Amal Feroui

Keys to Medical Imaging for healthcare professionals

Amal Feroui

Keys to Medical Imaging for healthcare professionals

Radiology and Computed Tomography

ScienciaScripts

Imprint

Any brand names and product names mentioned in this book are subject to trademark, brand or patent protection and are trademarks or registered trademarks of their respective holders. The use of brand names, product names, common names, trade names, product descriptions etc. even without a particular marking in this work is in no way to be construed to mean that such names may be regarded as unrestricted in respect of trademark and brand protection legislation and could thus be used by anyone.

Cover image: www.ingimage.com

This book is a translation from the original published under ISBN 978-620-6-69924-8.

Publisher:
Sciencia Scripts
is a trademark of
Dodo Books Indian Ocean Ltd. and OmniScriptum S.R.L publishing group

120 High Road, East Finchley, London, N2 9ED, United Kingdom
Str. Armeneasca 28/1, office 1, Chisinau MD-2012, Republic of Moldova, Europe
Printed at: see last page
ISBN: 978-620-7-01135-3

Keys to Medical Imaging for healthcare professionals

Radiology and Computed Tomography

Foreword

Bringing a book to fruition is a journey lasting several years of our lives, during which we learn, evolve, come across new knowledge, and sometimes reach the end of our patience. A book is in fact the fruit of several years' research. The great interest of the present book lies in the fact that it provides a solid grounding in the two main techniques of medical imaging: conventional and digital radiology, as well as classic and modern computed tomography. These modalities are increasingly used to help diagnose a wide range of diseases. The book covers the physical principle of X-rays, as well as the various systems for acquiring and reconstructing medical images.

General introduction

Medical imaging has revolutionized medicine, providing effective diagnosis in all areas of medical science. The investigation of the human body using images used to rely essentially on radiological examination. Today, the diagnostician has an arsenal of techniques at his or her disposal, including conventional and digital radiology, computed tomography, ultrasound, magnetic resonance imaging and scintigraphy. In medical imaging, the quality of image acquisition and interpretation determines the accuracy of diagnosis. The emergence of increasingly powerful computers has had a huge impact on medical image acquisition. They perform multi-faceted functions, such as controlling imaging equipment, transmitting, storing, visualizing, automatically extracting information, reconstructing and post-processing image data...etc.

The aim of this document is to review the main aspects of two medical imaging modalities: conventional and digital radiology, and computed tomography (CT). We present their schematic diagrams, their clinical applications and their respective places in the medical imaging market. We will also look at the different acquisition systems used to obtain quality images, on the one hand, and to aid diagnosis, on the other.

With all these considerations in mind, we have set seven objectives:
1. Understand the principle of medical imaging.
2. Learn about the different types and formats of images.
3. Learn about the main medical imaging modalities and their history.
4. learn the physical principles of medical imaging techniques (production of X-rays).
5. Understand the steps involved in image reconstruction.
6. Learn about image quality factors.
7. Understand procedures for using X-ray imaging devices.

Table of contents

Chapter 1
Medical imaging

Introduction

The last century has seen dazzling medical progress. The human body now holds virtually no secrets for medicine. Since the turn of the century, invention after invention, progress after progress, this wish has been fulfilled thanks to a number of new technologies, based on more or less recent physical principles. Medical imaging is, in fact, one of the areas of medicine that has seen the most progress over the last twenty years. In this 1er chapter, we define medical imaging and its history, then review its role in medicine and the benefits of computerized medical image processing. The different types of images and imaging are presented. We then describe the different modalities of medical imaging. Finally, a general overview of the most commonly used image formats will be presented.

I.   Medical imaging

Medical imaging encompasses all the techniques involved in creating a visual representation of the body, its organs, bones... without harming them. Since its very beginnings, medical imaging has undergone numerous evolutions, and thanks to new technologies, it has enabled considerable progress in our understanding of the human body, medical diagnosis and disease treatment. It encompasses the means of acquiring and restoring images of the human body based on various physical phenomena such as X-ray absorption, nuclear magnetic resonance, ultrasound wave reflection or radioactivity, sometimes combined with optical imaging techniques such as endoscopy [1]. It has revolutionized medicine by providing immediate, reliable access to clinical diagnostic information, such as anatomical features, and even certain aspects of metabolism, such as organ function, blood flow.... etc.

I.1.Principle

The discovery of medical imaging has revolutionized medicine, making it possible to obtain a medical image revealing precise information on the functioning of an organ, such as the heart and its arteries, or any other organ requiring a diagnosis or surgical approach. What's more, the image can be viewed in 2D, 3D and even 4D, enabling doctors to explore the human body and make increasingly precise diagnoses. It uses a variety of physical principles (US, X-ray, NMR, gamma ray). Medical imaging compiles a wide range of data and information thanks to its different techniques, and makes exhaustive computerized management of this information part of its practice.

I.2.History

The great revolution in medical imaging began with Roentgen's discovery of X-rays (RX) in 1895 [1]. At the time, this physicist was studying cathode rays using a Crookes tube. While using this instrument, he noticed that it caused fluorescence (emission of light under the influence of radiation) of a screen placed two meters from the tube. He concluded that this phenomenon was caused by another, as yet unknown, type of radiation. He named it after the letter symbolizing the unknown in mathematics, the X-ray. These rays of unknown origin had the ability to pass through bodies opaque to light. The 1st image is of a human hand: that of Madame Roentgen (she had arthrosis!), and x-rays were immediately of interest in medicine, first for orthopedics, then for exploring the thorax and abdomen.

The introduction of contrast-enhanced examinations further broadened the scope of radiology from the 1950s onwards.

Considerable advances in computer technology have led to the reconstruction of cross-sectional images from multiple projections: this is what CT (computed tomography) or CAT (computed tomography) scanning was all about in 1972.

-Ultrasound first appeared in 1915, thanks to sonar technology developed by sailors.

-Magnetic resonance imaging (MRI) was born in 1945. The emergence and development of these new technologies have revolutionized radiology and medicine in general. The use of gamma rays in medicine came much later, with the invention of the gamma camera giving rise to scintigraphy in 1990.

II.   Medical image processing

Computer-aided medical image processing can be used in all phases of medical image acquisition and processing. In the first instance, IT is directly involved in the generation of certain types of image that could not otherwise be obtained, such as CT, MRI, etc. **On** the other hand, digital image processing is a necessary phase in establishing a better diagnosis. In this phase, image compression algorithms are applied to reduce storage volume, and image quality enhancement operations are carried out to reduce acquisition noise. IT is also involved in the extraction of parameters of clinical interest (surface measurements, distances, densities, etc.) in order to establish the correct classification of pathologies. Finally, images can be transferred between hospital structures for rapid consultation of several experts to establish a precise diagnostic and therapeutic decision.

III.   How do you distinguish between a pathological and a healthy image?

A pathology may appear on the image as :

- a difference between the form examined and the known form (e.g. stenosis = vascular narrowing)

- a local variation in the gray level of an organ.
- Abnormal contrast (too weak or too strong) between an organ and its neighbors.
- unusual texture (e.g. osteoporosis = a disease characterized by thinning and weakening of the bones).

IV.   Types of medical imaging

Medical imaging has evolved from morphological to functional imaging. In fact, types of imaging can be divided into 3 groups:

IV.1 Morphological or anatomical imaging

It is used to study the anatomy of various organs, whether hard, soft, immobile or moving, such as detecting fractures (conventional radiography) or monitoring fetal development (fetal ultrasound) (Figure I.1).

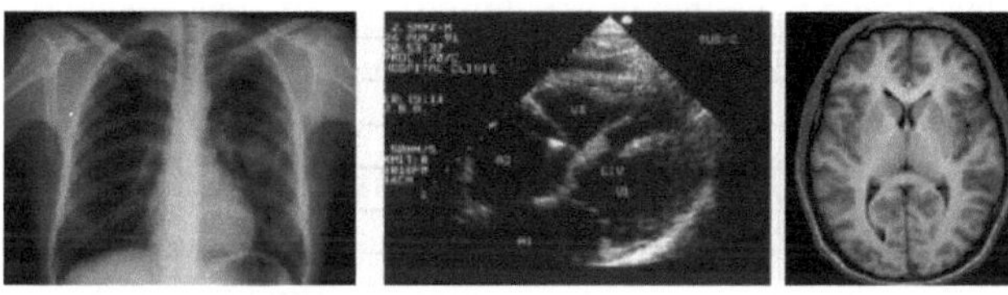

X-ray Ultrasound MRI

Figure. I.1. *Examples of morphological imaging.*

IV.2. Functional imaging

It is used to study organ function. It can detect dysfunctions preceding the appearance of morphological anomalies, and is therefore complementary to anatomical imaging (Figure I.2).

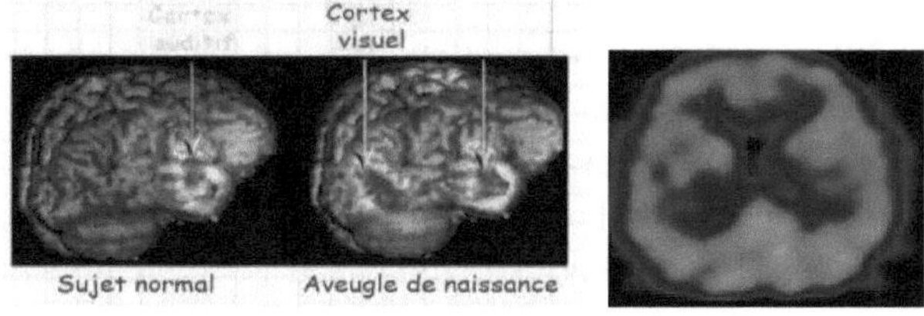

Scintigraphic images
Figure. I.2 *Examples of functional images*

IV.3. Molecular imaging

It can be used to visualize genes or proteins directly or indirectly. It is currently being developed mainly in small animals (Figure I.3).

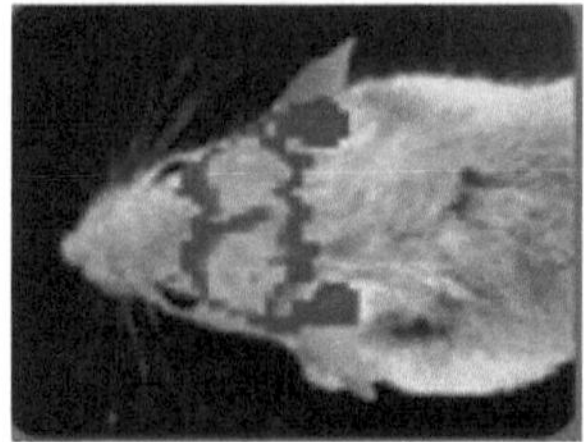

Figure I.3: Example of molecular imaging

V. General information on instrumentation techniques

In medical imaging, describes 4 main modalities

V.1. CT scanner

The basic principle is to scan an anatomical slice and acquire the X-ray transmission profiles in this slice, using an X-ray tube and detector [2]. The patient is placed on a table that moves longitudinally inside a short ring. Part of the incident radiation is absorbed by the tissues it passes through. The ring contains an X-ray tube which rotates around the patient. Detectors measure the residual intensity of the beam that has passed through the body. As the tube rotates, the incident and emerging X-rays captured are compared and converted into electrical signals. Complex computer processing then produces a reconstructed image of an axial section 1 to 10 millimeters thick on the screen. This image reflects variations in tissue absorption, with associated grey levels.

V.2. Ultrasound

Ultrasound is a medical diagnostic imaging technique that uses ultrasonic waves (US). US waves are acoustic waves with frequencies ranging from 20 kHz to 200 MHz, and their interest in imaging lies in their ability to propagate through tissues and reflect at interfaces between media with different US propagation characteristics. It is based on the emission of ultrasound by transducers, followed by reception of the echoes generated at interfaces and scattering centers [3]. Ultrasound is a widely used imaging technique, not only for imaging specialists, but also for obstetricians, cardiologists, urologists and, increasingly, general practitioners. The use of increasingly high-performance probes, the application of increasingly powerful image processing techniques and the introduction of 3D and 4D modes.

V.3. Magnetic resonance imaging

MRI is an imaging technique that combines *anatomical* and *functional* imaging. It provides both precise visualization of the structures examined, and lesion information about them. MRI uses the electromagnetic properties of the proton spins of hydrogen nuclei (subjected to an intense magnetic field and electromagnetic waves*)*. The hydrogen nucleus is present in all body tissues and fluids, and consists of a single proton. We liken these protons to small magnets which, in the absence of an external magnetic field, are animated by a rotational movement, randomly oriented in all directions. A *spinning* particle induces a microscopic elementary magnetic moment around it, aligned with its axis of rotation and represented by a magnetization vector. During an MRI scan, the body part under examination is placed in an intense magnetic field B0, which causes all free protons to align in the direction of this magnetic field [4]. The application of a specific amount of energy in the form of electromagnetic waves known as radiofrequency waves or pulses (RF) switches the orientation of these spins: this is excitation. When this interaction is interrupted, the spins tend to return to their equilibrium state. During relaxation, the protons emit signals that are picked up by the detector.

V.4. Nuclear medicine

Scintigraphy is an examination that evaluates the function of an organ such as the brain, heart, kidneys, lungs, thyroid or a body part such as bones or joints. Scintigraphy is a medical exploration technique that uses radioactive isotopes. It produces a medical image by detecting the radiation emitted by these isotopes after they have been captured by the organs to be examined. The technique involves injecting a radioactive product that can be identified by its temporary fixation on certain tissues or organs. The radioactive product is chosen according to the organ to be studied (lungs, bones, thyroid, heart, etc.) [5]. Once fixed, the doctor measures the radioactivity on the organ or tissues concerned using a device called a gamma camera.

V.   Image characteristics

An image is the representation of a scene, an object or a physical phenomenon acquired by a system such as: cameras, X-rays, scanners....etc.). The image can be defined as a two-variable function A (i, j) defined on a 2D (X-ray image...) or 3D (ultrasound image...) space. It can be in two forms: analog (photography, video...etc) or digital (image acquired, created, processed and stored by binary coding (computer-processed image)).

- (i, j) is the position of a point in space on the Projection plane
- A (i,j) is the intensity (or brightness) at the point with coordinates (i, j)
- digital image: is a 2D matrix where the elements are pixels.

V.1.Pixel

Is an image point. It is characterized by its position (i, j) and intensity value (color or grayscale (GS)) [6].

V.2.Greyscale (NG)

It is defined as the luminous intensity represented by each pixel of the image. It varies from 0 to 255 (0: black and 255: white) (Figure I.4).

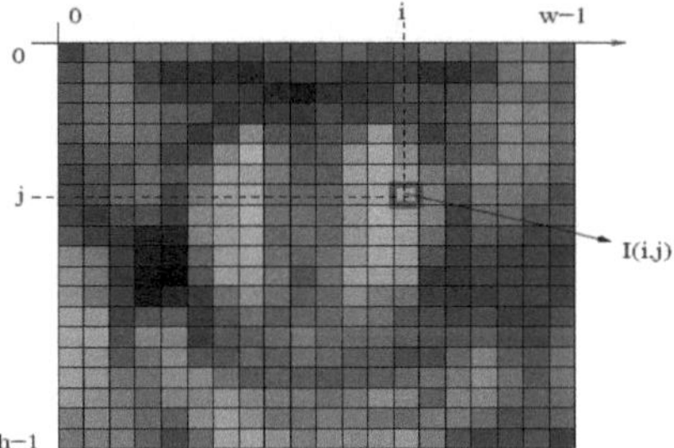

Figure I.4. grayscale *image.*

V.3.Luminance

Is a quantity corresponding to the visual sensation of luminosity of a surface (Figure I.5). Luminance is the average of all pixels in the image.

$$moy = \frac{1}{NM}\sum_{i=0}^{N-1}\sum_{j=0}^{M-1} A(i,j) \tag{I.1}$$

With : A (i,j) : original image, N : number of rows in the original image, M :number of columns

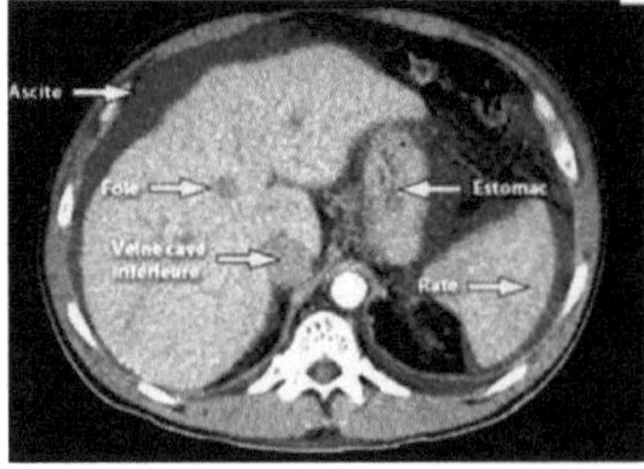

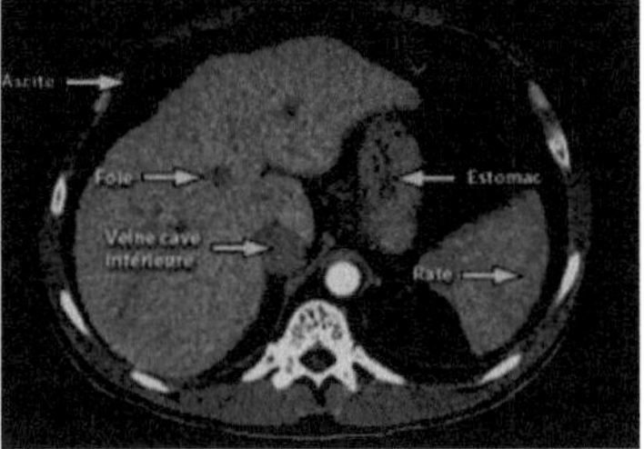

Figure I.5. *Example of luminance.*

V.4.Contrast

Is an intrinsic image property that quantifies the difference in brightness between the light and dark parts of an image (Figure I.6). Contrast is defined as follows:

- Standard deviation of greyscale variations

$$c = \sqrt{\frac{1}{NM}\sum_{i=0}^{N-1}\sum_{j=0}^{M-1}(A(i,j) - moy^2)}$$

(I.2)

- Variation between minimum and maximum grey levels

$$C = \frac{\max(A(i,j))-\min(A(i,j))}{\max(Af(i,j))+\min(A(i,j))}$$

(I.3)

Where: max: maximum NG value; min: minimum NG value.

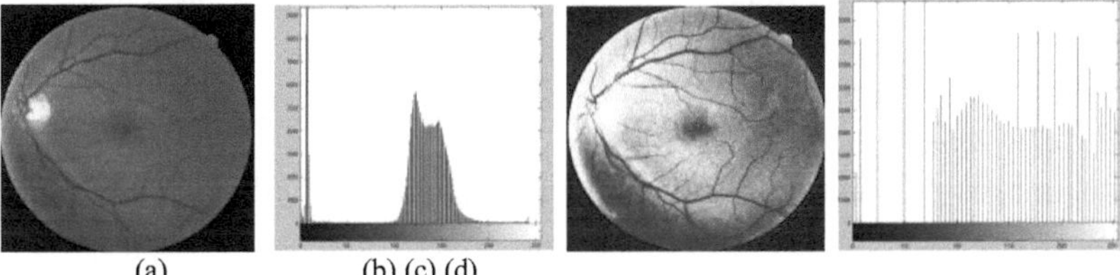

(a)   (b) (c) (d)

Figure I.6.*Example of image contrast;(a): low-contrast image;(b): histogram of Figure (a);(c): high-contrast image;(d): histogram of Figure (c).*

In figure (I.6), we can see that the dynamic range of the image is increased by extending the pixel values over all the NGs, so contrast is increased and the image content becomes more visible.

V.5. *Image resolution*

Is the number of pixels per unit length of the scanned structure (typically dpi (dots per inch)) (Figure I.7).

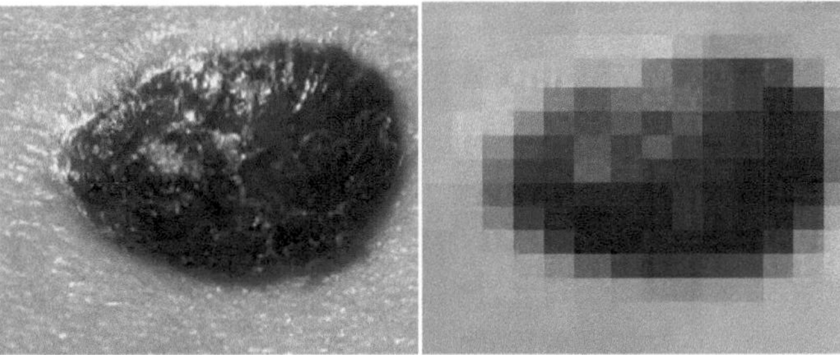

Figure I.7. *Image resolution*

VI.   Image types

VI.1.Binary images

Binary images are the simplest, called "Bichromes" (mostly black and white), and are ontologically digital (they can be coded and decoded directly to base 2) (Figure I.8).

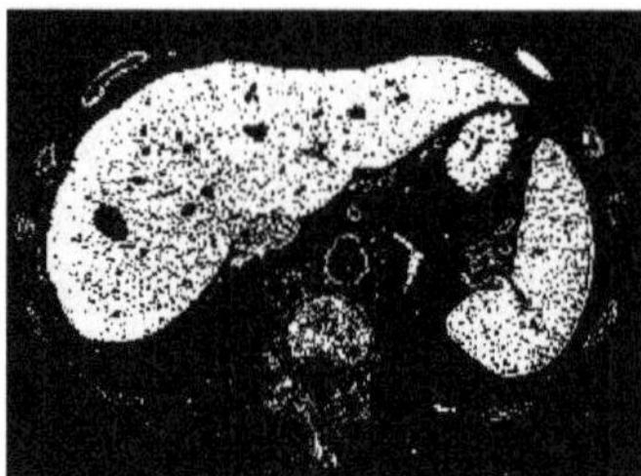

Fig. I.8.*Example of a binary image*

VI.2. grayscale images

In this case, gray levels range from 0 to 255. Zero represents black and 255 represents white, while 128 is the average gray level. This type of image is coded on 8 bits (Figure I.4).

VI.3 Color images (RGB)

Color images are images coded by three fundamental colors (red, green, blue), where each color is coded as a byte. It is of size (m, n,3) and can be interpreted as a stack of 3 arrays of size (m, n) defining the red, green and blue intensity of each pixel. Thus, the red intensity of pixel (10,10) in the RGB image is RGB (10, 10,1). The green intensity is given by RGB (10, 10,2) and the blue intensity by RGB (10,10 ,3).

R(i,j) and V(i,j) and B(i,j); the combination of these three types of plane gives the final color (Figure I.9).

Where; m: number of rows in the color image; n: number of columns in the color image.

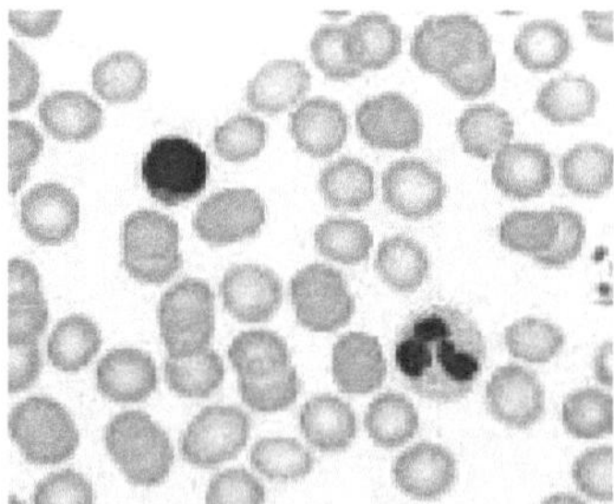

Fig. I.9.*Example of a color image*

VI.4.Indexed images

The indexed image is a color image. These colors are stored in a color table. This table is a matrix of n*3 (n number of colors), so the image is a matrix containing integers between 1 and n, with each n playing the role of an index relative to the color table.

VI.5.3D images

3D images represent a scene in three dimensions. The "pixel" is then called a voxel. This represents an elementary volume (Figure I.10).

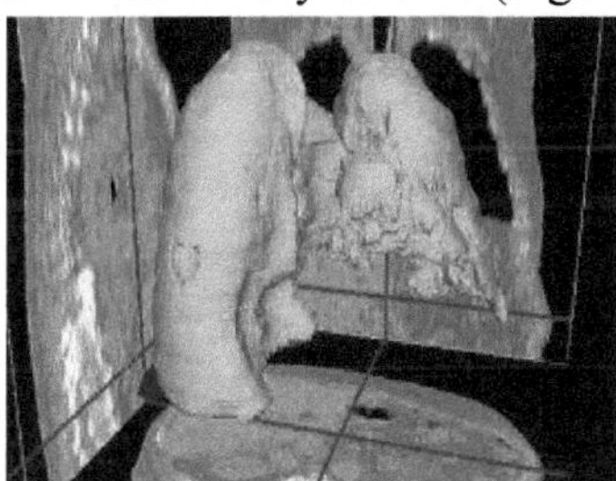

Figure. I.10. *Example of a 3D image.*

VII. Image format

An image can be saved in different formats.

VII.1 BMP (windows bitmap) format

BMP is the format developed by Windows. The main advantage of this technology is the quality of the images supplied: no compression, i.e. no loss of quality. However, this makes it a very heavy image format (large file size), which is rarely used on the Internet [7].

VII.2 JPEG format (joint photographic experts group)

This is the most common format (extension **.jpg**), developed by photographers to transmit images of professional photographic quality. JPEG images are 24-bit images. In other words, they can display a spectrum of 16 million colors. This is the best image quality available. This format is ideal for large images. It is currently the most widely used image compression format on the market, and offers the advantage of an adjustable compression ratio. However, care must be taken not to select too high a compression ratio, otherwise the image will become unusable (resulting in a loss of information and therefore a visible loss of quality if the compression ratio is high).

VII.3 GIF (graphics interchange format)

The GIF color palette comprises around 16 million colors, but can only display between 2 and 256 in the same image, making the file size more or less small. For this reason, the GIF format should not be used for photographs requiring a large number of color nuances. This format is used for logos, wallpapers, black-and-white photos, etc. It allows you to have a transparent background, i.e. to superimpose one image on another while allowing the background image to show through, which is what has made it so popular. It can also be used to create animations. It contains several sequential images within the same file.

VII.4. PNG (portable network graphics) format

This image format was created to replace the GIF, but is little known to the general public. Yet it is one of the most powerful. It combines almost all the advantages of JPEG with those of GIF. It reaches 16 million colors (like JPEG), but also allows total or partial transparency of part of the image (like GIF).

VII.6. TIFF (tagged image file format)

The TIFF format is a non-destructive, uncompressed file format widely used by many image processing programs. It is supported by all operating systems, including Windows and Linux. It can work in most color spaces, such as RGB. Its many advantages make it a preferred format for printing or digital photography, but its heavy weight makes it unsuitable for web use. It produces a very high quality image, but has a large file size. Nevertheless, TIFF allows the use of lossy (JPEG) or lossless data compression algorithms.

V.7. DICOM (digital imaging and communications in medicine) format

The DICOM standard was issued by the ACR (American College of Radiology) in association with the NEMA (National Electrical Manufacturers Association). It is used by most manufacturers of medical imaging equipment. The DICOM file contains textual information about the patient (name, age, weight, etc.), the examination performed (region explored, etc.), the technique used (scanner, MRI, etc.) and the raw data (uncompressed form). This absence of compression is often desirable, as it simplifies transfers and enables information to be preserved in its native, easy-to-decode form.

Conclusion

In this chapter, we have presented the aspects needed to understand the importance of medical imaging in medicine, firstly, the definition of medical imaging, the different types of images and their properties have been described, then a general overview of medical imaging modalities has been presented, we have ended this chapter with a description of image formats and some exercises.

Exercises

Exercie1

Consider the following image A(i, j) :

200	0	0	12	5
200	59	50	36	5
59	59	50	45	36
12	128	45	16	16
200	128	64	5	36

1. What is the size of image A?
2. How many bits are used in this image?
3. How many grey levels are there in image A?
4. What is the relationship between the number of bits and quantization?
5. Draw the histogram?
6. Find out if :
- the histogram of image A is concentrated on low grey levels?
- Histogram h is concentrated on high gray levels?

Average value of a region R : $\mu = \frac{1}{m*n} \sum_i^m \sum_j^n T(i, j)$

Variance of a region R : $\sigma^2 = \frac{1}{m*n} \sum_i^m \sum_j^n (T(i, j) - \mu)^2$

7. Calculate mean and variance.

Exercise.2

1. What's the difference between a color image and an indexed image?
2. What are the advantages and disadvantages of the GIF format used in medical imaging?
3. Why are morphological and functional imaging complementary?
4. In the images below, indicate :

4.1. Type of imaging (justify your answer) ?

4.2. The acquisition technique in Figure 3 and 4 and briefly explain their principle?

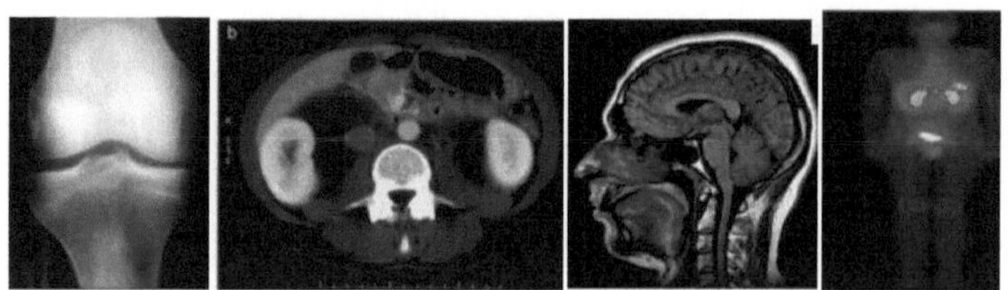

Fig.1 fig.2 fig.3 fig.4

Chapter 2

X-ray imaging

Introduction

The great revolution in medical imaging began in 1895 with Roentgen's discovery of X-rays [1]. This discovery gave birth to a medical specialty (X-ray imaging). X-rays have many applications in physics, biology and medicine. This chapter is devoted to presenting the physical basis of X-rays. We describe the phases of X-ray production and the various components of an X-ray tube. We then present the law of X-ray attenuation. At the end of the chapter, the biological effects of X-rays are studied.

I.   Electromagnetic waves

Radiation is the process of emitting or transmitting energy in the form of electromagnetic waves. An electromagnetic radiation (or wave) consists of the propagation of an electric field E and a magnetic field B perpendicular to each other. These fields oscillate in phase and are themselves perpendicular to the direction of propagation. A sinusoidal electromagnetic wave is characterized by its frequency of vibration and its amplitude.

The amount of energy (E) carried by electromagnetic radiation is:

$$E = h\,\nu \; (h : \text{is Planck's constant } (h=6.62\ 10\text{-}34\ J.s). \quad \text{(II.1)}$$

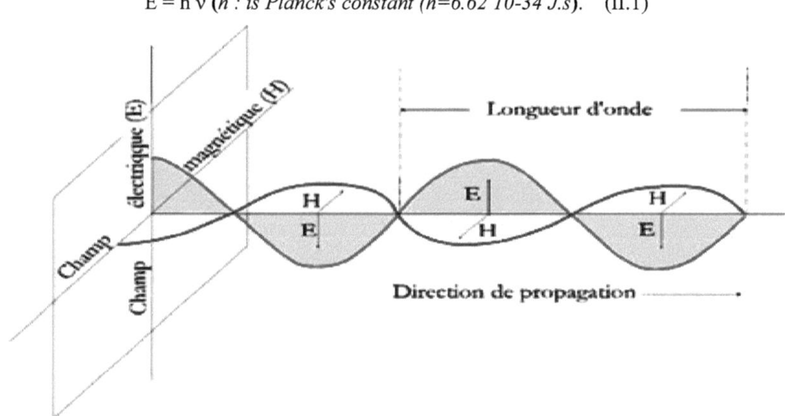

Figure II.1: *Electromagnetic wave*

Electromagnetic waves travel in a straight line, in a vacuum or in matter, with a constant speed in the same medium. As they travel through matter, they may interact with the atoms in the medium through which they pass, resulting in absorption, scattering or reflection of the initial wave.

I.1. Electromagnetic spectrum

Represents the distribution of radiation intensity as a function of frequency (figure II.2). It includes radiation with very different properties and uses, from radio waves to cosmic rays. The visible spectrum is very narrow. The colors correspond to different wavelengths [8].

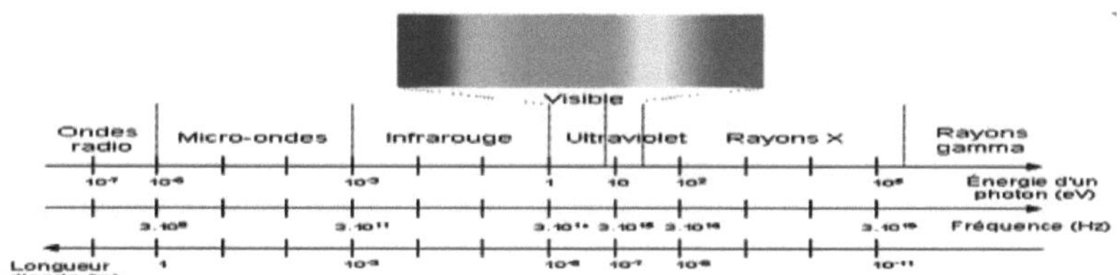

Figure II.2: *Electromagnetic spectrum*

X-rays are part of the electromagnetic radiation family, along with light, microwaves, radio waves and γ-rays. X-rays are electromagnetic radiation of shorter wavelength (higher frequency) than light. They have enough energy to eject an electron when they are absorbed or deflected (ionizing radiation).

Electromagnetic radiation in excess of 10 KeV is ionizing radiation, and as such is considered dangerous. Imaging examinations using X-rays (radiography and tomodensitometry) and γ-rays (scintigraphy) are accompanied by precautionary measures and are governed by regulations designed to limit health risks.

II. X-ray production

This radiation is emitted as follows (Figure II.3): A vacuum is created in a glass enclosure. A target called the anode (+) is bombarded by a beam of electrons accelerated by a high potential difference. The electrons are obtained by heating a filament called the cathode. The cathode consists of a metal filament heated by the passage of a current of a few milliamperes. The current provides mobile electrons that are easily accelerated by applying a high potential difference between cathode and anode (around 450 kilovolts for the most common generators) [9].

The electron bombardment surface on the anode is called the focus. The surface of the anode is oblique to the direction of the electron beam, allowing the X-rays to exit the tube. X-ray tubes are subject to severe thermal and mechanical stresses, which can reduce the speed of clinical examinations and render certain protocols unusable for a certain period of time (while the system cools down). To limit this effect, the rotating anode tube has been introduced. Other developments, such as the possibility of using two focal points at the anode from the same filament, have improved spatial resolution.

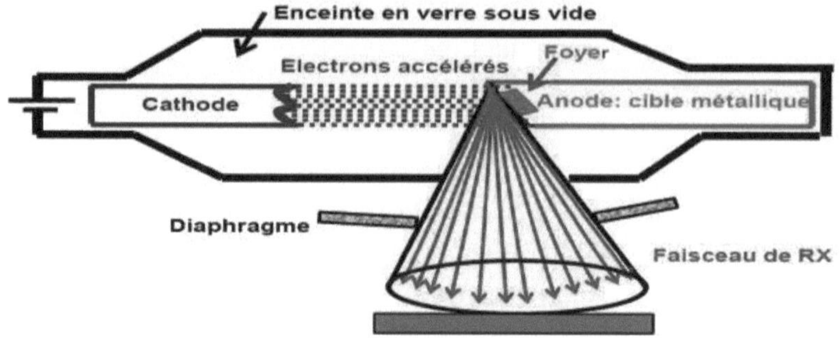

Figure II.3. *Diagram of an X-ray tube*

III Interaction of electrons with matter

Electrons are light particles carrying an elementary electric charge, negative for negatons and positive for positrons. When positrons move through a material medium, they lose their kinetic energy through interactions with the atoms of the medium they pass through. They interact either with the electrons of the atoms making up the medium, or with their nuclei.

Two mechanisms are responsible for the formation of X-rays in an X-ray tube: general emission (or bremsstrahlung) and characteristic emission. In both cases, X-rays result from the interaction between a stream of electrons launched at high speed onto a material target.

III.1 Electron interaction with an atomic electron (characteristic emission)

Characteristic emission is a minor phenomenon in X-ray production.

Two mechanisms can occur when electrons interact with the atom's electrons:

III.1.1 Ionization

If the energy of the incident electron is greater than the binding energy (E>30 eV) of the atomic electron. Incident electron collides with an electron in the fundamental **K** orbital of a tungsten atom. The incident electron has therefore just collided with an electron from a deep layer (often K) and manages to eject it. The hole left is quickly filled by the passage of an electron from a more peripheral layer (L, M, N ,O, P) towards the incomplete deep layer, releasing energy in the form of an X-ray (fluorescence). This shift is due to differences in binding energy between the electron layers.

Any electron falling to the K level from any higher level (L, M, N, O, P) releases an energy of between 57.4 keV and 69.5 keV [10].

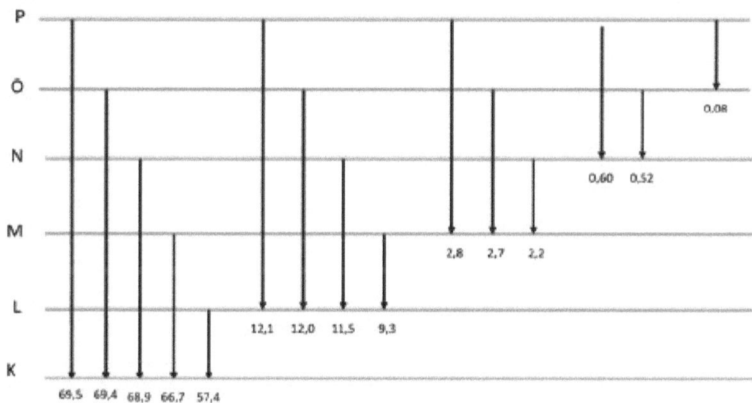

Figure II.4. *X-ray energy released for each electron layer*

III.1.2 Excitation

If the energy transferred by the incident electron is equal to the difference between the binding energies of the two electron layers of the target atom, the atomic electron jumps to an orbit corresponding to a less-bound electron layer, and is said to be excited.

- The atomic electrons concerned are the weakly bound electrons of the outer layers (
Figure II.5.)[10].

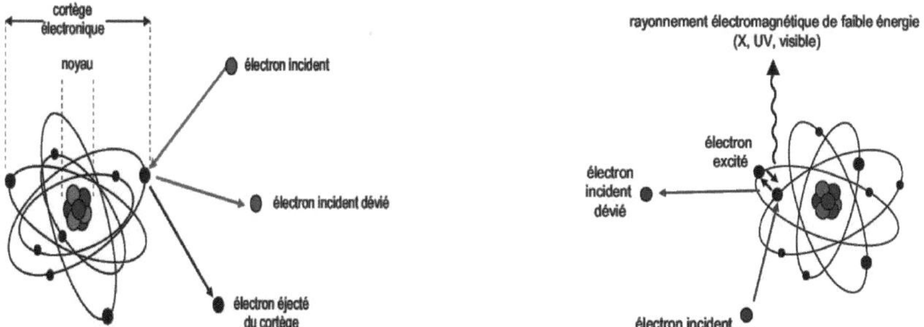

Figure II.5.*Ionization and excitation phenomena respectively.*

III.1.3 Fluorescence

During ionization or excitation. The electron seeks to return to its original energy level. When it returns to its original layer, energy is released in the form of an X-ray whose energy value depends on the difference between the two energy levels. As the binding energy of electrons is unique for each layer and each atom, the energy spectrum of the X-rays emitted is characteristic of the atom in question. It is an emission whose energy depends solely on the target atom (figure II.6).

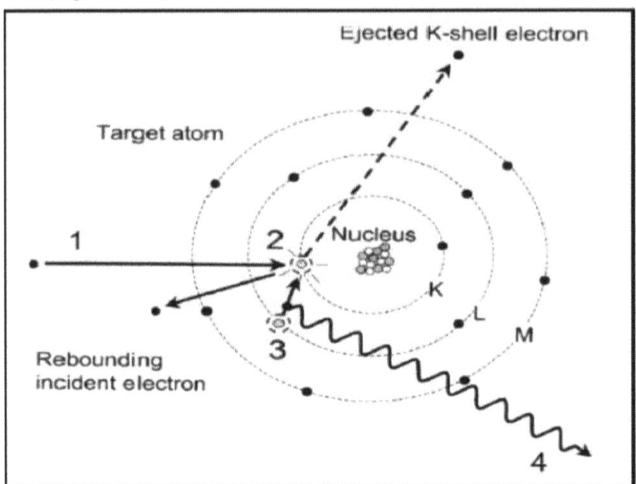

Figure II.6.*Fluorescence phenomenon*

III.2 Interaction of electrons with the atomic nucleus (general emission)

General emission is the main mode of X-ray formation in radiology. General emission occurs when the electron passes close to the nucleus and is attracted by its charge. The electron is deflected and slowed down (figure II.7).
The resulting loss of energy is reflected in the emission of one or more X-rays.

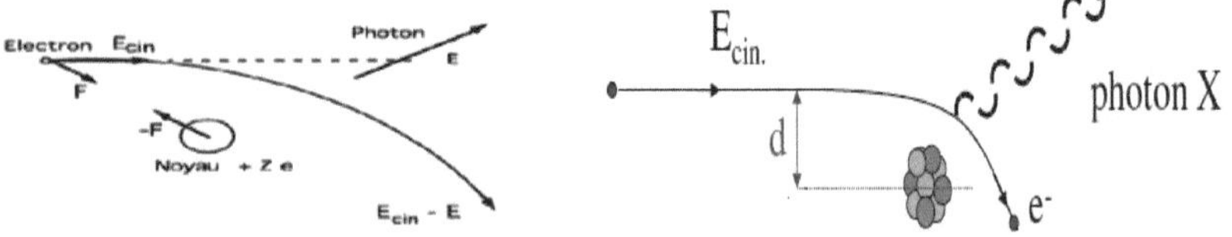

Figure II.7. *Braking radiation*

The electrons gradually lose their energy along their entire trajectory. They are deflected into the coulombic field of the target atom. This manifests itself as slowing or braking. The energy lost is emitted in the form of braking X-rays. The energy of the X-rays produced in this way is variable.

X-ray energy depends on 3 parameters:

1. Kinetic energy of the electron

2. The attraction of the nucleus, i.e. its charge (Z)

3. The distance between the electron and the nucleus, which is random.

In this process, the incident electron can lose all its kinetic energy E_{cin} at once, giving an upper limit to the frequency of the emitted photon (continuous spectrum). The frequency depends solely on the acceleration voltage and not on the metal of the target.

Braking obviously depends on how close the electron is to the nucleus, and the photons emitted can have any energy between zero kinetic energy and E_{cin} .

The probability of producing a high-energy x-ray is lower than the probability of producing a low-energy x-ray. The emission spectrum therefore decreases with energy, with a roughly linear decay [11].

IV. X-ray spectrum

The quantity of X-rays produced in a radio tube depends on :

(1) The number of electrons thrown at the target,

(2) Their kinetic energy (for general emission)

(3) Core size.

An X-ray emission spectrum is the superposition of a continuous spectrum and a discrete spectrum of lines.

IV.1 Continuous spectrum

The continuous spectrum corresponds to braking radiation (Bremstrahlung). It is due to the interaction of incident electrons with the nuclei of target atoms. The shape of the continuous spectrum is shown in Fig. II.8. It shows that the spectrum decreases towards higher energies. As a result, low-energy photons are the most numerous. The incident electron can lose all its kinetic energy $(E\ )_{cin}$ at once, giving an upper limit to the frequency of the emitted photon.

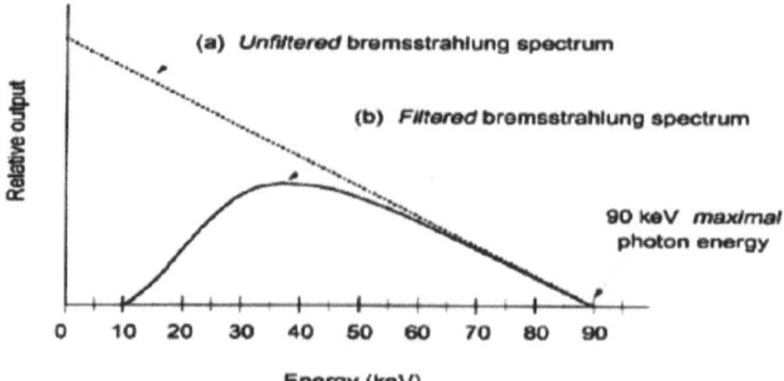

Figure. II.8. *Continuous spectrum;(a) : Spectrum without filtration of very low-energy photons;(b) : Spectrum with filtration of very low-energy photons.*

IV.2 Line spectrum

The line spectrum corresponds to the energy distribution of the fluorescence photons characteristic of the electronic rearrangement of the target atoms after interaction (excitation or ionization) between the incident electron and an electron from the inner layers of the procession (Figure II.9). Figure (II.9) shows the emission spectrum of tungsten at two acceleration voltages: 50 kV and 90 kV. It can be seen that 50 kV is not sufficient to reach the K layer of tungsten.

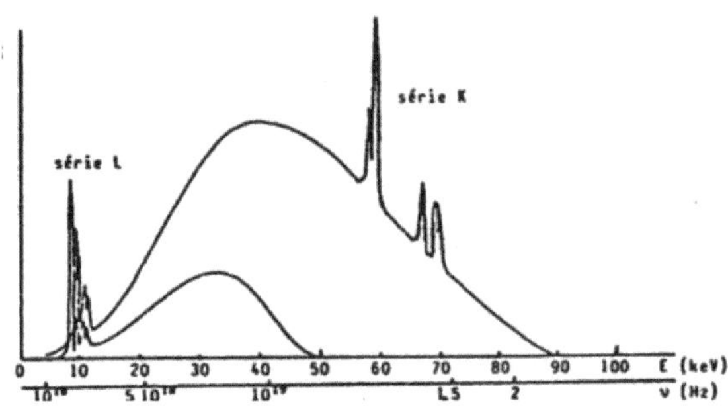

Figure II. II.9.*Line spectrum.*

IV.3 Combined spectrum

The atom used in the majority of X-ray tubes used in radiodiagnostics is tungsten (W). The majority of X-rays are produced by general emission, whose energy varies between 0 and the kinetic energy of electrons, and whose relative quantity varies inversely with their energy. Low-energy X-rays are quickly stopped by the materials surrounding the target, and are excluded from the useful beam leaving the tube. Figure (II.10) shows the combined X-ray spectrum. It can be seen that the photon flux is made up of a low-energy background and characteristic lines from the higher-energy K-layer. The tube's efficiency is very low: 1% of X-rays versus 99% of heat.

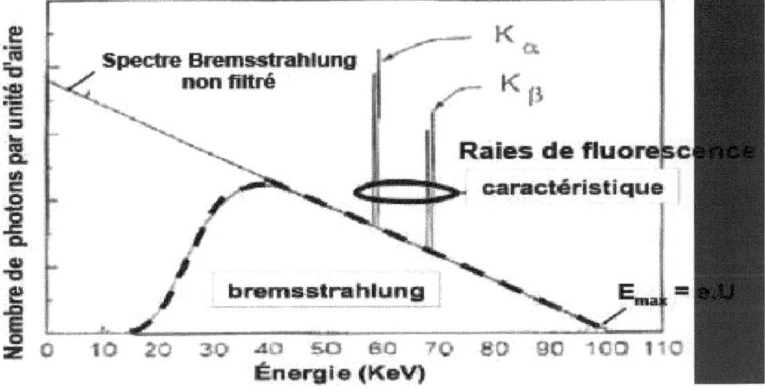

Figure II.10. *Spectrum at RX*

V. X-ray tube technology

The X-ray tube consists of several components, as shown in figure II.11.

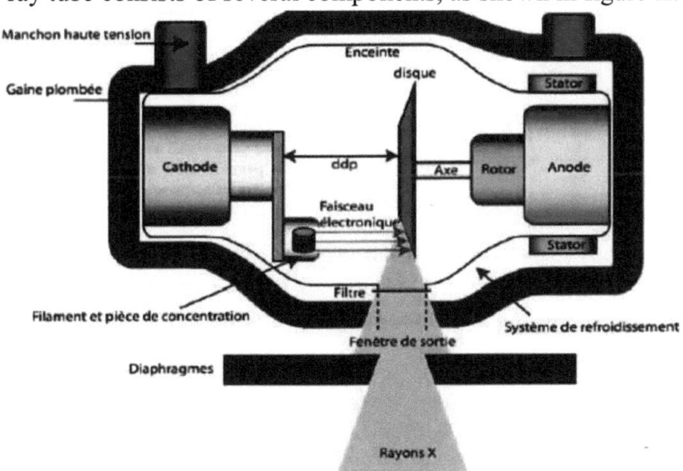

Figure II.11. *X-ray tube*

In the following section, we describe the various components of an X-ray tube.

V.1. cathode

The cathode consists of

- one or two filaments to create an electron source.
- a concentrator that holds the filaments in place.

V.1.1. Filament

This is a helical winding of wire with a cross-section of 0.2 to 0.3 mm. A high-intensity heating current flows through it. The intensity of this heating current is regulated to the extent that the potential difference between cathode and anode is sufficient. In most cases, the cathode carries two windings of different sizes, arranged side by side or in line with each other. In this case, the heating current is carried by three conductors (Figure II.12.). The filaments are characterized by :

- High melting temperature (melting point 3422°C)
- Good heat conduction

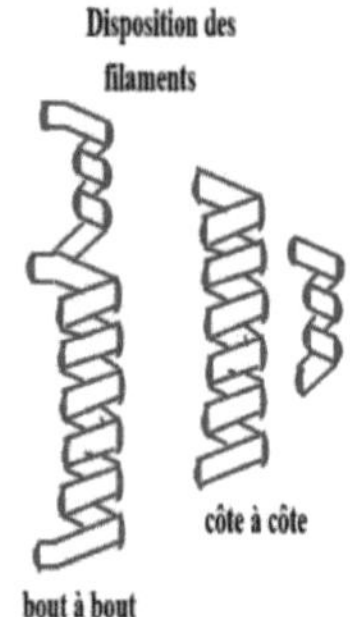

Figure II.12. *The cathode*

V.1.2. Concentration piece

It's a metal part with a bowl shape. The filaments are placed at the bottom. Its role is to :

- It prevents filament deformation.
- Focuses electrons on the anode.
- Determine the shape of the focus. (figure II .13).

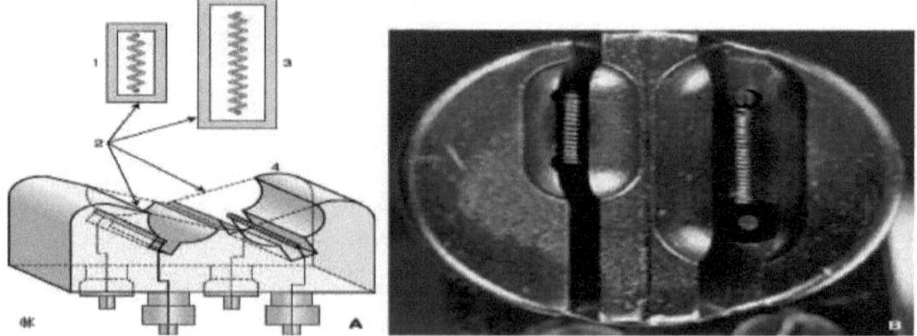

Figure II.13. *Filament and focuser with two foci*

V.2. Anode

Its design takes into account two imperatives: high power and a small X-ray production area. It is an essential component of the X-ray tube. It must meet three criteria:
- Be sufficiently dense (high Z) to promote X-ray production.
- High melting point to withstand high temperatures.
- Good thermal conductivity for rapid heat dissipation.
There are two types of anode: fixed and rotating.

V.2.1. Fixed anode

It's limited in power, simpler (less expensive). It's a tungsten plate set in a copper cylinder, placed opposite the cathode to be hit by the electron beam and placed opposite the cathode. The copper cylinder is extended outside the glass tube by a radiator to ensure heat dissipation. The surface of the anode hit by the electrons, called the electron focus, is rectangular (figure II.14).

To reduce the apparent surface area of the focus, visible from the tube's emergence window, the tungsten plate is oblique to the electron beam: perpendicular to the electron flow, the focus is seen as a shortened square. This apparent surface is called the optical focus. The anode angle, i.e. the angle between the track and the director beam (the median part of the X-ray beam), varies between 10° and 20°.

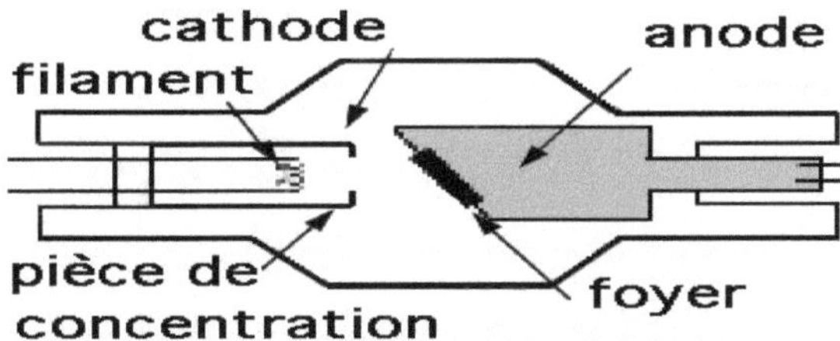

Figure II.14. *Schematic diagram of a fixed anode.*

V.2.2. Rotating anode

Rotating anodes are used in medium- and high-power tubes. They consist of a rotor-stator pair, a transmission shaft and a disc. The rotating anode has the shape of a flattened truncated disk, a few millimeters thick, rotating opposite the cathode: the electron beam strikes it on its peripheral part, the tungsten anode track whose orientation is oblique in relation to the electron beam. This disk is supported by a shaft integral with a rotor mounted on ball bearings, and rotates during electron bombardment at high speed: 3,000 rpm (Figure II.15).

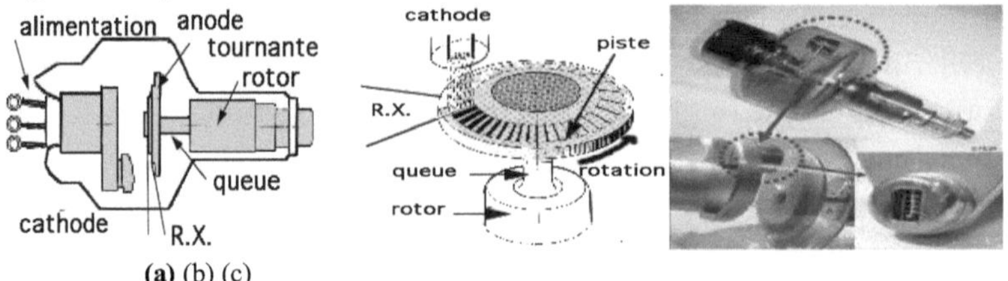

(a) (b) (c)

Figure II.15. *(a and b): Rotating anode; (c): Diagram of a **rotating** anode tube*

V.2.3. Molybdenum anode

It is used in mammography tubes: hit by 30 KeV electrons, it produces 17, 20 KV X-rays, since the photoelectric effect is predominant. In these tubes, the need for excellent resolution, especially under magnification conditions, dictates the use of small foci (0.1-0.3mm).

V.3. Bulb (enclosure)

The enclosure contains the anode and cathode, and is designed to maintain a high vacuum (so that the movement of the electrodes encounters no obstacles), and is made of glass (radio-transparent). This bulb, placed in insulating oil, is usually made of glass, which is a good electrical insulator, is transparent to thermal radiation and welds perfectly to the metal of the electrodes. Unfortunately, this glass slightly attenuates X-rays at the emergence window [12].

V.4. Cooling system

A cold water piping system or fan cools the oil surrounding the tube (figure II.16).

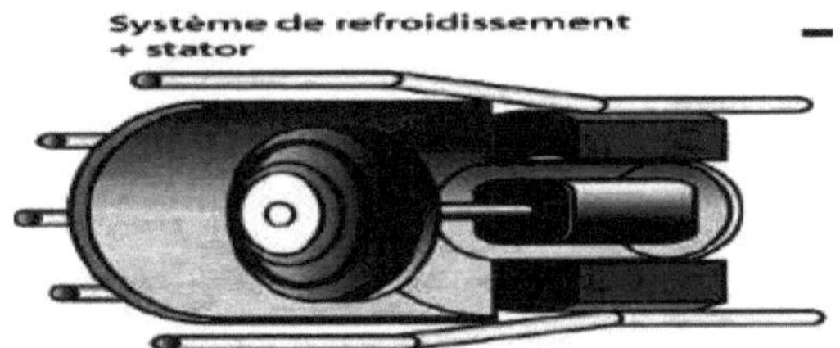

Figure II.16. Cooling system

V.5. Sheath

The leaded sheath is a 3 to 5mm envelope placed inside a metal cylinder lined with lead except for the exit window (figure II.17). The sheath insulates the exterior from heat, high voltage and stray X-rays. An exit window is placed opposite the anode to allow X-rays to pass through. It contains an insulating oil and an expansion compensating device to prevent expansion.

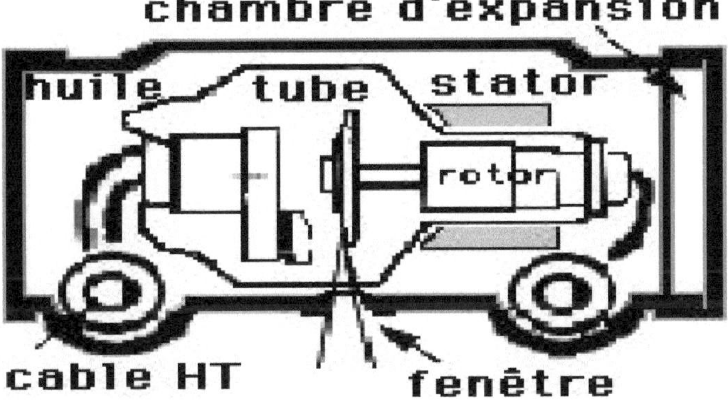

Figure II.17. *Diagram of the tube in its sheath*

V.6. Filter

The filter is placed against the output window. It homogenizes the energy of the X-ray beam by eliminating low-energy photons.

V.7. Diaphragm

These are metal strips placed on either side of the exit window. They determine the (rectangular) irradiation field and limit scattered radiation.

VI. Interaction of X-rays with matter

Two main ways in which X-ray photons interact with matter: the photoelectric effect and the Compton effect

VI.1 Photoelectric effect

The photon collides with an electron in the atom's inner layers. The energy of the incident photon is transferred to the electron, which is ejected from its layer. Some of this energy is used to extract the inner electron (binding energy); the excess energy is found in the form of kinetic energy (E_{cin}) of the ejected electron. The photoelectric effect can only occur if the energy of the incident photon is greater than the binding energy of the electron. The kinetic energy of the photoelectron is ultimately transferred to the medium in subsequent ionizations. The atom's return to its ground state is accompanied by energy emission in the form of a fluorescence photon.

The fluorescence photon is emitted when an electron from the upper layers takes the place left vacant by the ejected electron, with the emission of an electron (figure II.18) [13].

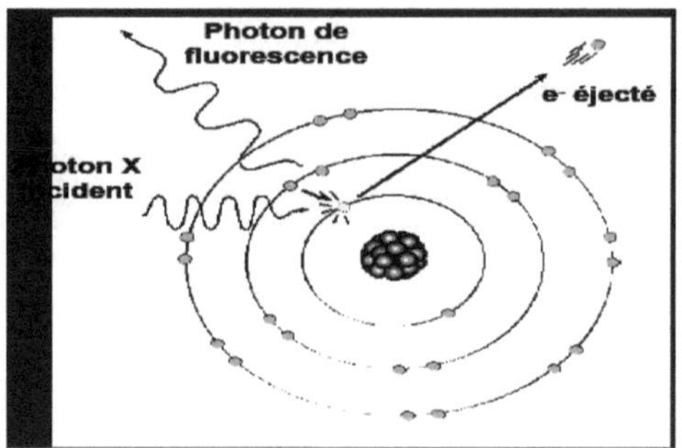

Figure II.18. *Photoelectric effect*

VI.2 Compton Effect

The photon collides with a free or weakly bound electron, to which it gives up some of its energy. A photon of lower energy is scattered in a direction different from the initial direction (Figure.II.19). The compton scattering coefficient varies little with the atomic number of the material, and practically depends on the mass of material present per unit area. The loss of the photon's initial direction produces a scattering blur in the radiant image. The compton effect concerns atomic electrons belonging to loosely bound electronic layers.

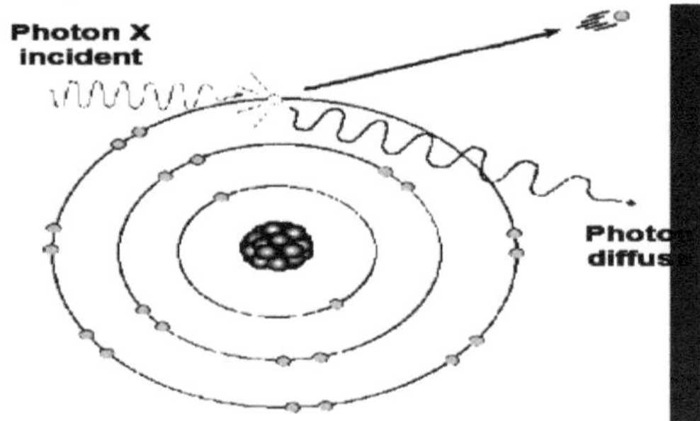

Figure II.19.*Compton effect: This is the scattering of a photon by an electron.*

VII. X-ray attenuation law

A unidirectional beam of monoenergetic photons passes through a material screen. Let I(x) be the intensity of the beam (number of photons crossing the unit area normal to the beam per unit time) at position x (Figure.II.20). Let's call -dI the intensity variation over an infinitely small thickness dx. Knowing that -dI is proportional to the incident intensity and the thickness x.

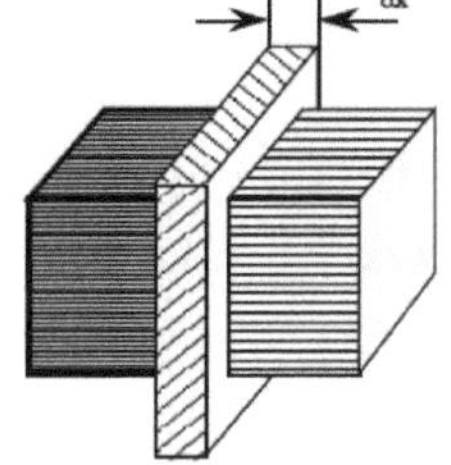

$$-dI = \mu(E, M)I(x)dx. \qquad II.1$$

The proportionality coefficient $\mu(E,M)$, known as the linear attenuation coefficient, depends on the energy E of the incident photons and the medium M. It has the dimension of the inverse of a length. Integration of equation (II.1) gives the attenuation law for a monoenergetic parallel beam of electromagnetic radiation as a function of thickness x :

$$I(x) = I_0\, e^{-\mu(E, M)x}$$

With I(x): the intensity of the beam after passing through a thickness x of material, I_0: the intensity of the incident beam: $I_0 = I(x = 0)$. The intensity of electromagnetic radiation decreases exponentially as a function of the thickness of material traversed. The attenuation coefficient varies greatly as a function of the material and photon energy. Generally speaking, it increases with the atomic number of the medium and decreases with the energy of the radiation [14].

VIII. Biological effects of X-rays

The ionization energy of the main atoms of biological interest is between 11 and 14 eV. X-rays (10 and 150 keV). The biological effects of ionizing radiation are the end result of physical events produced by the radiation in the living environment. The very brief passage of a photon (or ionizing particle) causes excitations and ionizations that trigger a succession of physico-chemical reactions that can lead to changes in cellular and then tissue functions and structures. Quantitatively, the energy absorbed, or the number of ionizations in relation to the number of molecules, remains excessively low, but it is sufficient to cause lesions that can be significant.

- At the molecular level: Ionizing radiation affects DNA, causing varying degrees of cellular damage.
- At cellular level: Either the DNA molecule is capable of self-repair, and there will be no cellular repercussions. Or it is incapable of doing so, and this can lead to mutations within the cell, or even cell death.

Cells are all the more sensitive because they are poorly differentiated and divide rapidly.

VIII.1 Effects of X-rays on the body

Ionizing radiation has two different types of effect on the body.

VIII.1.1 Non-stochastic effects

They appear when the dose received reaches or exceeds a certain value; there is therefore a threshold below which these effects do not appear.

VIII.1.2 Stochastic (or random) effects

Occur only in certain individuals, apparently at random, in an irradiated population. These include the induction of cancer or malformations in offspring. There seems to be no threshold; even low doses can trigger these effects. They are delayed and their severity is independent of the dose received. However, the frequency with which stochastic effects appear is dose-dependent.

Conclusion

In this chapter, the physical basis of X-rays is presented. The origins of X-ray production and the various components of an X-ray tube were studied. The chapter concludes with a presentation of the biological effects of X-rays.

Exercises

Exercise.1

The emission of an X-ray photon by a metal is due to certain electronic transitions between two energy levels and to the interaction of the electron with the nucleus of an atom. The energy level diagram for molybdenum is shown below.

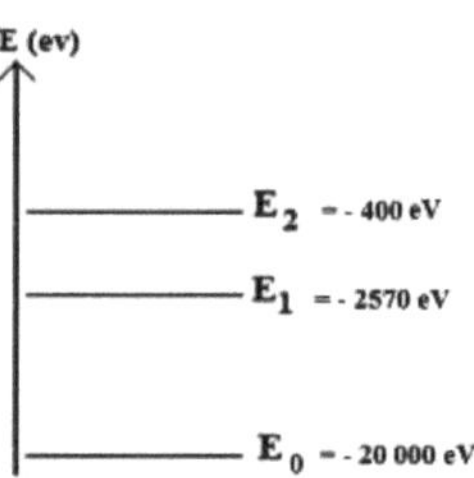

2. Indicate all the possible transitions that are accompanied by the emission of a photon?
3. Calculate, in electron volts (eV), the energy variations corresponding to these transitions...
4. Which of the transitions considered produces the X photon associated with X-radiation? Why?
5. What are the different parameters influencing the energy emitted by an X-ray?

Exercise.2

Consider the figure shown in figure 1:

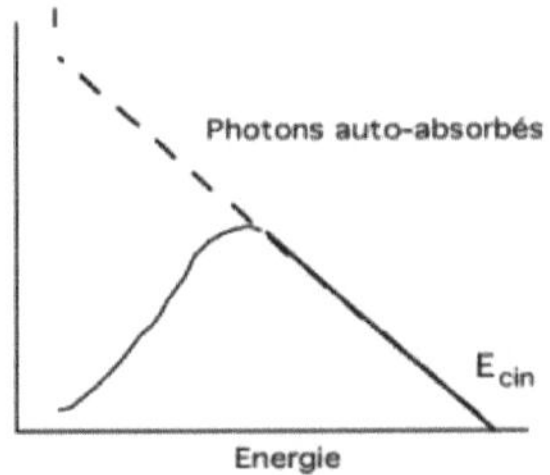

1. Explain the shape of the figure?
2. Explain how the current generated by the filament and the voltages generated by the generator affect the quality and quantity of x-rays generated by the X-ray tube.
3. How should the anode be constructed to produce X-rays?
4. What's the point of using two hearths in the rotating anode?

Chapter 3

Conventional and digital radiology

Introduction

X-ray radiography was born of the discovery of X-rays by German physicist Wilhelm Conrad Ronghen in November 1895. This discovery was quickly followed by the first clinical application, in January 1896.

In 1913, Coolidge invented the X-ray tube, which led to the rapid development of X-ray radiography using photographic plates. This technique is very useful for visualizing bone structures and abnormally dense masses that particularly absorb X-rays. However, it only provides a projected image, and therefore does not allow in-depth visualization in the direction of observation. Today, traditional X-ray radiography has evolved by digitizing the acquisition image. This makes it easier to manipulate and save images on computerized equipment. In this chapter, we focus on presenting the principle of conventional and digital radiology. In the first section of the chapter, we describe the radiology chain, as well as the factors that influence the quality of the X-ray image. We then present the acquisition systems used in conventional radiology. In the second section of the chapter, we describe the advantages of digital radiology and its detection systems.

I.   X-ray chain

The radiographic chain is made up of a series of instruments and equipment, all of which play their part in image quality (Figure III.1). Like all chains, if one link breaks, the whole chain ceases to function. It is advisable to check that the system is working properly, either periodically or when a recurring defect is observed on the X-ray images. To carry out an X-ray, you need to :

- A generator powering the X-ray tube
- An X-ray tube
- A filter that makes radiation spectra narrow and monochromatic.
- Diaphragm to delimit the X-ray beam,
- Primary collimation to reduce scattered radiation.
- A detection system that converts X-ray photons into an electrical signal.

In the following paragraph, we describe the role of the various components in the radiological chain.

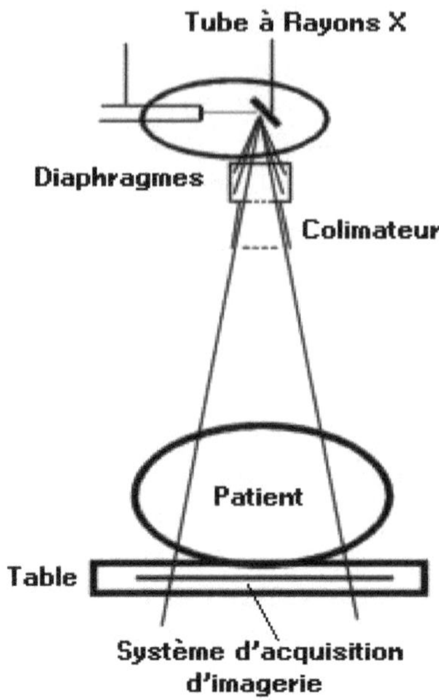

Figure III.1: *X-ray chain*

I.1. X-ray generator

The X-ray generator houses all the circuits supplying the X-ray tube. It is connected to the tube by electrical cables. The X-ray generator comprises two main circuits:
- The low-voltage circuit that powers the filament
- The high-voltage circuit for high potential difference

The generator can also be used to :
- Transform low-voltage alternating current into high-voltage direct current
- Adjust filament heating intensity
- Determine exposure time.

I.2 X-ray tube

X-ray tubes are devices for producing X-rays. Whatever the type of tube, X-rays are generated according to the same principle. A high electrical voltage (of the order of 20 to 400 kV) is established between two electrodes. This generates a flow of electrons from the cathode to the anode. The electrons are slowed down by the target atoms, producing continuous braking radiation, part of whose spectrum is in the X-ray range. These electrons excite the target atoms, which re-emit characteristic X-ray radiation through the phenomenon of X-ray fluorescence. The spectrum leaving the tube is therefore the superposition of the braking radiation and the target's X-ray fluorescence. X-ray tubes have extremely poor energy efficiency, with most of the electrical power (99%) dissipated as heat. Tubes must therefore be cooled, usually by circulating water, an oil bath or a rotating anode system.

I.3. Filter

We generally use 2mm aluminum filters for voltages from 60 to 120 kV, and 2mm copper and aluminum filters for voltages above 120kV.

I.4. Diaphragm

The diaphragm is used to cleanly delimit the size and shape of the X-ray beam exiting the tube. Originally, it was a simple, calibrated opening, usually rounded, in a lead plate that was attached to the tube sheath by means of a slide. Today, the most widely used radiodiagnostic system consists of two stages of lead shutters, movable inside a metal box and adjusted either manually or by remote control. This delimits a rectangular opening, materialized by a luminous area visualizing the zone to be radiographed (luminous diaphragm). For X-rays, radiotherapy uses thick shutters and a device known as a "collimator".

I.5. Collimator

Collimation reduces scattered radiation and protects patients from excessive irradiation

I.6. Detection systems

In some indirect systems, the information relating to the detector's exposure to photons is contained in the form of a latent (virtual) image. The detector must undergo a specific operation to transform this latent image into a real image. More modern, direct systems can instantly transform the information received by the detector into an image. In section V, we present the different types of detectors used in radiology.

II. Radiant image formation

The X-ray beam emitted by the tube is homogeneous. This beam passes through the human body, which absorbs a portion of the X-ray radiation proportional to the thickness, density and atomic number of the zone it passes through. The X-ray beam is thus unevenly attenuated, and becomes heterogeneous as it leaves the body. It thus carries a radiant image, which is transformed into a luminous image by a detector (figure III.2).

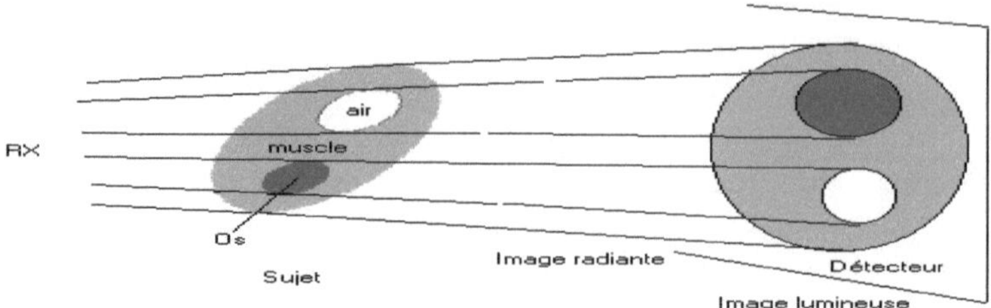

Figure III.2: *Radiant image formation*

III. X-ray image quality factors

Radiological image quality is judged on several parameters: contrast, sharpness, incidence and centering. In the following paragraph, we describe these parameters in detail.

III.1 Contrast

It represents the difference between black and white areas on the print. It depends on the technical conditions under which the image was taken, and on the observer's visual acuity. It is the measurable difference in relative intensity between two points of light. The contrast in the image is due to the difference in attenuation between water, air and bone, at low energy values [15]. If an X-ray beam of intensity I passes through the same thickness d of two homogeneous media 1 and 2, it will be unevenly attenuated by the body and will emerge heterogeneous with different intensities I1 and I2 depending on the media through which it passes. This is the radiant image: not visible to the eye. To quantify this difference: the notion of radiological contrast (figure III.3).

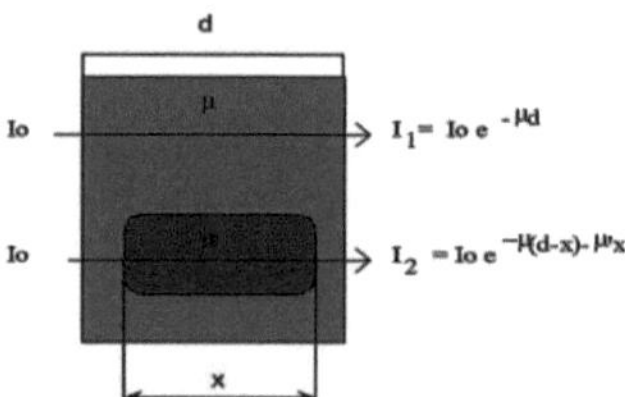

$$I_1 = I_0 e^{-\mu d}$$

$$I_2 = I_0 e^{-\mu(d-x)-\mu'x}$$

Figure III.3. *The contrast*

The contrast between two points of the radiant image with respective intensities I1 and I2 is :

$$C = I1-I2/ (I1+I2) \quad III.1$$

Very low-energy X-rays cannot be used when the thickness is great. Because of their high attenuation, the amount of incident radiation must be high to ensure that sufficient radiation is still transmitted through the patient.

The contrast is directly related to the acceleration voltage (E) and the difference in attenuation coefficients, which depends on the quality of the radiation and the nature of the media (Figure III.4).

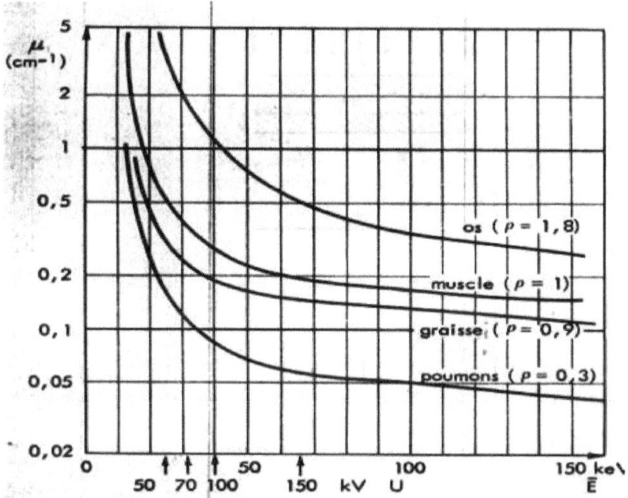

Figure III.4. *Relationship between applied voltage and attenuation coefficient*

As the voltage applied to the tube increases, the energy of the photons increases, so □□diminue and the rays are more penetrating. Above 100 Kvolts, there is virtually no change in □□en as a function of energy. However, whatever the E, we have : □os > □eau > □air and their relative values evolve as a function of the voltage applied to the tube. As a result, you need to choose a compromise between high contrast and low dose. The value of E is adjusted empirically (with experience) for each type of examination.

Low- to medium-penetration X-rays provide contrast-rich images (figure III.5). This type of radiation is used in particular for bone radiographs: the contrast between the bone (which is white) and the soft tissues is maximal. Similarly, this is the zone of maximum absorption for iodine

41

contrast agents, used to opacify the urinary tract, bile ducts and vessels (figure III.6).

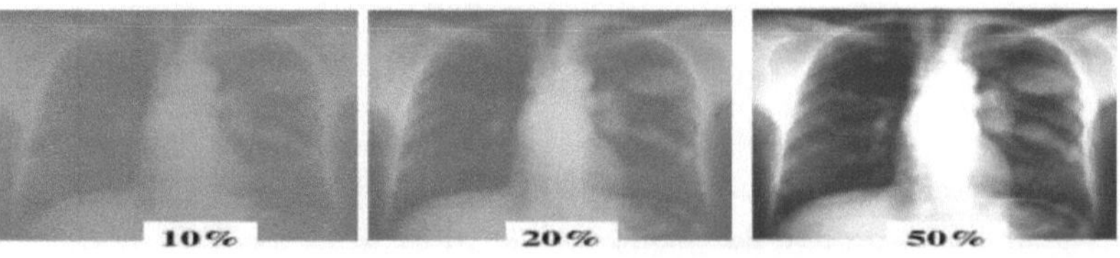

Figure III.5.*Variable contrast images*

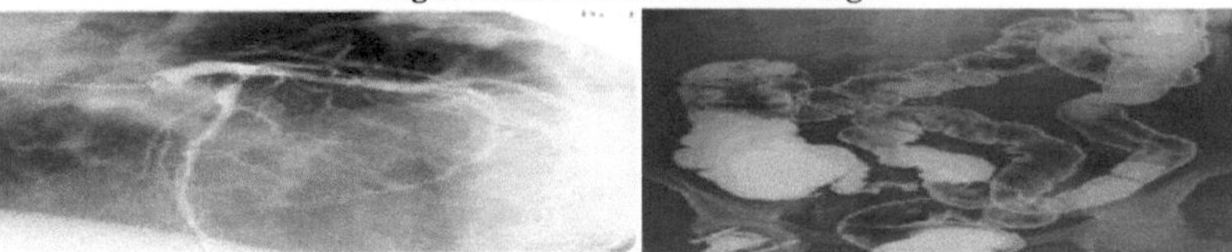

Figure III.6.*Use of contrast medium.*

III.2. Sharpness

The image should be sharp, with no blurring and well-defined contours.

III.3. Impact

Anatomical analysis requires comparison with images taken in a defined reference position.

III.4.Centering

The useful image must be at the center of a film of minimal size.

IV. Factors in radiological image degradation

The contours of the image must be sharp (perfectly delineated); a precise line separates opaque dark and light areas. The absence of sharpness is blur, a defect that we strive to reduce.

IV.1 Scattered Radiation Blur

The attenuation of the X-ray beam in the human body produces scattered radiation, which can "shower" the X-ray film in a uniform manner, removing all contrast from the image.

This type of blurring is a quantitatively important parameter in radiology: attenuation by diffusion is 4 to 5.5 times greater than that by absorption (photoelectric).

The blurring of scattered radiation poses several problems

- Unnecessary irradiation (of nursing staff in particular).
- contrast reduction in radiography.

To reduce scattered radiation, it is necessary to :

- Reduce the volume irradiated, using a diaphragm or localizers on the primary radiation, or by compressing the explored region to reduce its thickness;
- The use of an anti-scatter grid to select the primary radiation by its direction, stopping rays from different directions. The grid is made up of thin lead strips separated by a medium transparent to X-rays. The primary beam passes through the blades of the grid, while the scattered radiation, in a different direction, is stopped by the blades.

To prevent scattered radiation from reaching the manipulator, a shield is used.

IV.2 Magnification blur

A radiograph is a conical projection on which anatomical elements are superimposed and appear distorted (figure III.17). The magnification G is expressed as

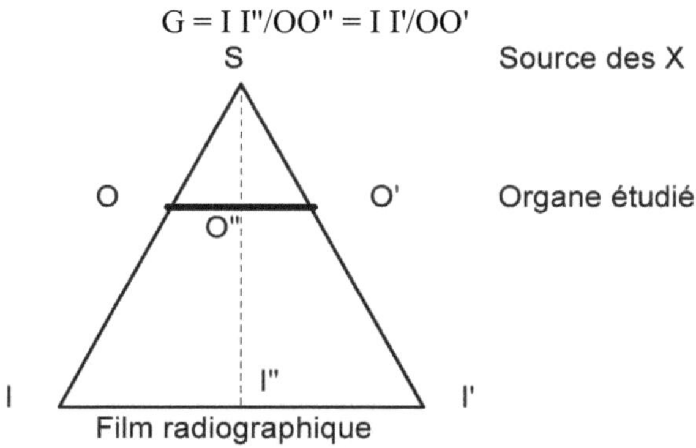

Figure III.7. *Magnification blur*

Given that sin(OSO") = II"/SI = OO"/SO, the magnification G is expressed as follows:

$$G = SI / SO$$

As a result, magnification increases overall when the film is moved further away from the X-ray source (SI increases).

IV.3 Kinetic Blur

The patient breathes, the heart beats, the digestive organs move, and muscular immobility cannot be controlled for long.

This is the most worrying blur. The moving anatomical element moves at a speed that can be considerable (instantaneous speed reaching 100 to 200 mm/second). The length of time covered depends on the exposure time. This blur can be reduced by :

- immobility; short exposure time; rapid sequence of shots: 50 to 100 fps.

IV.4 Receiver blur

The receiver has a granular structure: silver bromide grains in the film, luminescent grains in the intensifying screen or luminance amplifier, and even the matrix structure of a digitized system. An ideal straight boundary line therefore translates into an irregular line, and therefore into imprecise contours. The quality of the receiver's spatial resolution therefore determines the degree of image sharpness.

V. Detection systems in conventional radiology

In conventional radiology, images are acquired using a combination of film and intensifying screen, placed inside a cassette. In this section of the chapter, we describe the various components of X-ray film and intensifying screens.

V.1. X-ray film

In radiology, , photographic film is used in two ways , firstly as an X-ray detector, and secondly as an image recorder .

The radiographic film consists of :

1. Substrate: made of triacetate or polyester, approx. 200 microns thick;

2. Intermediate layer to ensure adhesion between substrate and emulsion

3. Emulsion: X-ray sensitive element , composed of a mixture of gelatin, silver bromide , and various correctors , gelatin silver bromide . It forms a layer very close to 30 microns thick [16].

The emulsion is usually distributed on both sides of the film (two-layer film) or on one side only (single-layer film).

Monolayer films feature an opaque antihalation layer on the side opposite the emulsion to prevent radiation reverberation. They provide better spatial resolution and are used in mammography).

4. a protective surface layer: This is permeable to treatment fluids acting on the emulsion, while providing mechanical protection.

However, the film remains fragile. Fingerprints (false images of calcifications in mammography) should be avoided. Films are best stored vertically, to avoid crushing the emulsion.

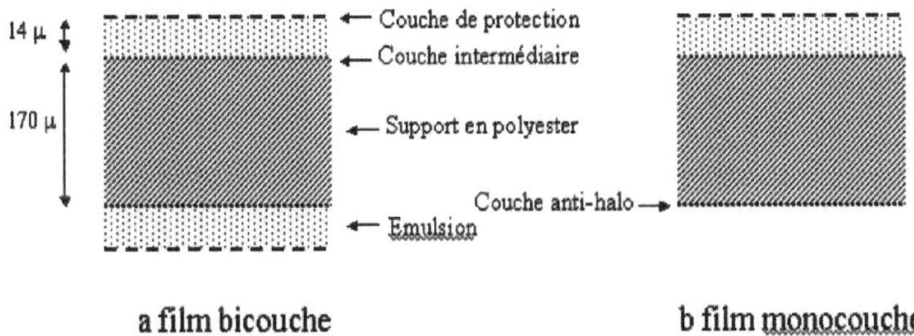

Figure III.8 X-ray film structure [16].

V.2. Reinforcing screens

X-ray film is not very sensitive to X-rays, and a significant amount of X-rays is required to achieve adequate film darkening. To increase the effectiveness of the X-ray film, it is usually placed between two intensifying screens in a cassette. To reduce irradiation, intensifying screens are placed in contact with the film. These are luminescent structures that emit light under the action of X-rays, which impress the emulsion and reinforce the action of the X-rays (Figure III.9).

The reinforcing screens are formed :
- A white, light-reflecting plastic base,
- A thin layer of luminescent crystals, excited by X-rays and giving off light in the form of luminous photons.
- A colorless, antistatic protective layer. It is washable, and should be cleaned regularly, particularly in mammography, where dust can simulate
  micro-calcifications. If double-layer films are used, the cassette will contain two reinforcing screens, positioned in contact with each side of the film. When using single-layer films, the screen is placed in the cassette in contact with the emulsion (rear side of the film).

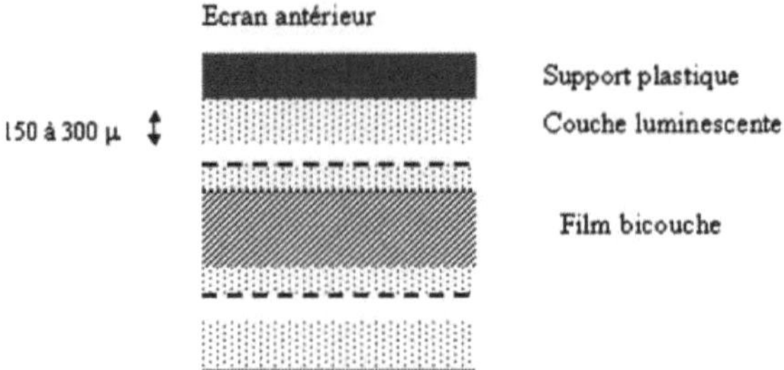

Figure III.9. *Layout of the screen-film pair* [16].

V.3. Cassette

The X-ray film is placed inside the cassette between the two screens (Figure.III.10). The cassette is simply a closed enclosure shielding the film from daylight and containing two intensifying screens placed on either side of the film. It has an X-ray-transparent front face made of aluminum or plastic, and a rear face containing a thin lead plate to attenuate direct radiation and stop backscattered radiation. Cassette size varies from 15x30cm to 43x35cm according to an international medical standard. The cassette opening-closing system depends on the processor used, as darkrooms with manual development have all but disappeared in favor of full-day systems with automatic development.

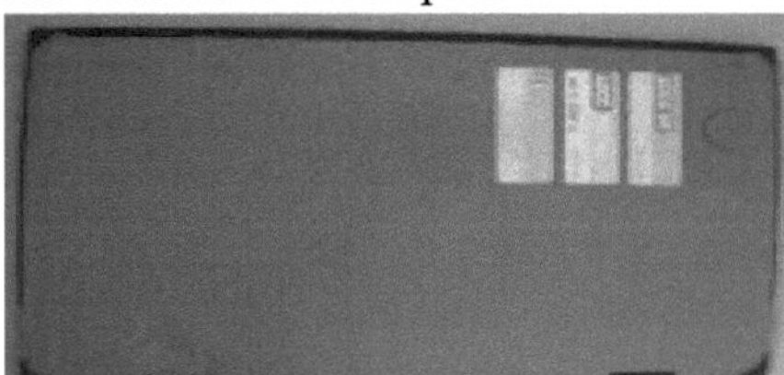

Figure III.10. *Cassette*

VI. Image formation radiology

In conventional radiology, image formation takes place in two stages: latent image formation and development.

VI.1 Formation of the latent image

The film is imprinted by light . This effect cannot be detected physically: the image is said to be latent. It is revealed by chemical processing . Photons hitting the silver bromide grains dissociate them , by photoelectric effect (pulling an electron from the Br- ion, which becomes a Br atom) , into bromine and silver atoms . 5 to 6 such dissociations in a single crystal (i.e. a million atoms) will constitute the latent image for this crystal, which will persist until development, when each one will constitute a development nucleus. The phases in the formation of the X-ray image are illustrated in figure III.11.

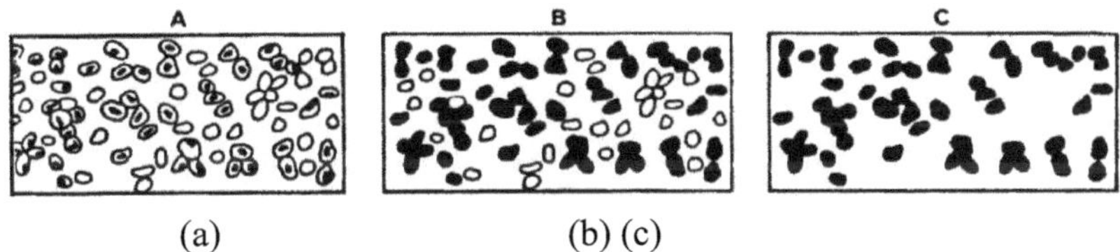

(a)   (b) (c)

Figure III.11. Stages of image formation.

- Figure (III.11.a) shows, after exposure, silver bromide grains that have received X-rays or light carry a latent image .
Figure (III.11.b) shows that after the use of a developer, latent image-bearing crystals are transformed into metallic silver.
- Figure (III.11.c), shows that in the fixative, unexposed crystals are eliminated . Areas sensitized by X-rays will appear black. This darkening is more intense the greater the quantity of X-rays received.

VI.2. Development

X-ray film development takes place in 4 or 5 phases, and can be manual or automatic.

VI.2.1.Manual development

In a darkroom, the film is taken from the cassette , fixed at all four corners to a frame which stretches and stiffens it. This frame is successively immersed , for specific lengths of time, in the following baths: developer (5 minutes), intermediate wash (very brief) , fixer (10 minutes), final wash (20 minutes) , then dried in the open air or in a stream of hot air .

VI.2.2.Automatic development

All automatic processors use the same method . The film, taken from the cassette in the dark placed at the processor's inlet , is driven by a cascade of rollers successively through the 3 tanks (developer , fixing, washing) , and then through a dryer (hot air or infrared) . The entire treatment may take 90 or 120 seconds at a temperature of around 35° (Figure.III.12).

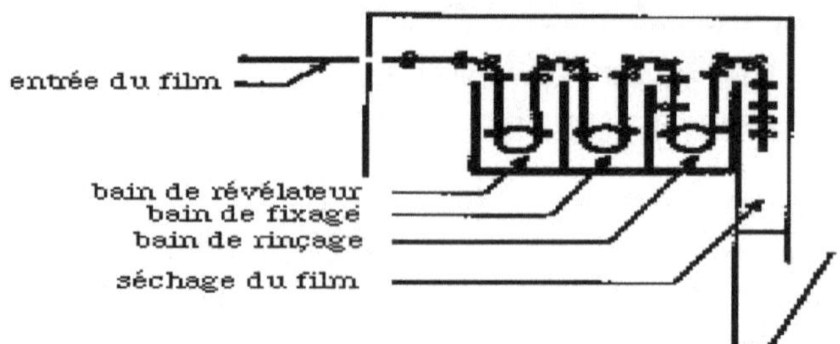

Figure III.12. *Sectional drawing of a developing machine .*

VII. Limits of conventional radiology

Conventional radiology has a number of disadvantages in medical imaging:
1. The information received on the photo receiver is frozen and can no longer be modified.
2. Film storage: Film ages under the effect of temperature and humidity, resulting in increased base fog and loss of sensitivity or contrast.
3. Cost of chemical consumables for development.
4. The image obtained continuously and in real time is coarse and not very bright.

VIII. Digital radiology

Digital radiology is replacing conventional radiology. It provides high-resolution images, helping to improve medical diagnosis, while subjecting patients and the body to low levels of X-ray exposure. Digitized X-ray examinations use not only an X-ray tube, but also a computer system responsible for document acquisition and processing. Digital collection of the X-ray image takes place in several stages (Figure.III.13)
1. detection: the radiant image is received by a detector (which replaces the film-screen pair), giving rise to an analog signal
2. analog-to-digital signal conversion
3. digital signal processing
4. digital-to-analog signal conversion on display console

The digital image lends itself to computer processing:
1. image display on a screen
2. Contrast modification through processing operations.
3. Improved visibility.

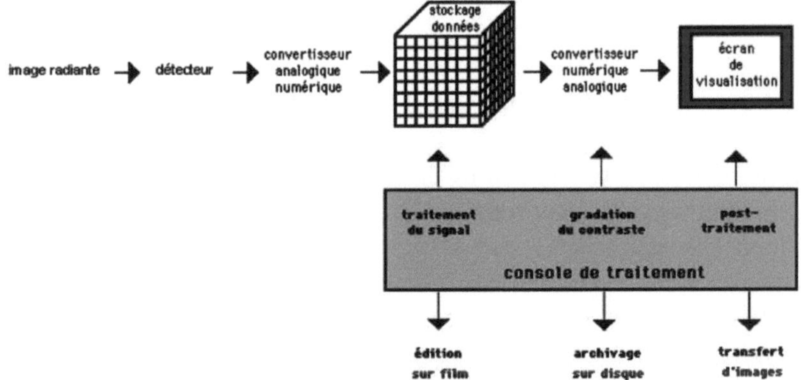

Figure III.13._C hate digital radiology_

VIII.1 Advantages of digital radiology

Digital imaging continues to develop, making it possible for doctors:
- a more reliable diagnosis.
- access information at any time, on site or remotely, archived and stored on media (hard disk, USB, CD...etc.), transmitted via secure networks or consulted directly on screen: which is fast, economical and environmentally friendly.
- reduce exposure to X-rays or minimize irradiation and comply with radiation protection standards.

VIII.2. detection systems

In digital radiology, there are two types of detectors for collecting the radiant image:

- Scanning detectors: image intensifier tube, memory screens, selenium drum. The radiant image is received on a flat (memory screens or image intensifier tube luminance amplifier) or slightly curved (selenium drum) support. To obtain a digitizable electrical signal, the latent image must be scanned.
- Or with a camera (image intensifier tube)
- Laser beam (memory screens)
- Or by electrometer strip (drum)
- Matrix planar detectors: the electrical signal generated within the detector is collected point by point on an active matrix.

In this section of the chapter, we describe the operating principle of the different types of detectors used in digital radiology.

49

VIII.2.1.Luminance amplifier-TV camera

This type of detector is not new: in the 60s, it enabled the development of televised radioscopy, followed by digital angiography. The amplifier is an electronic tube placed between two screens and subjected to an electrical voltage. The input screen receives the weakly luminescent X-ray image and transforms it into a stream of electrons inside the tube. The electrical voltage applied to the tube accelerates the electrons, which bombard the second screen with additional energy. The output screen transforms the electron stream into visible light, restoring the image with a considerable gain in brightness. The fluoroscopic image is then retransmitted on a TV screen. The system consists of two converter screens and a vacuum tube [17] (Figure.III.14).

- Vacuum tube

It accelerates electrons without interaction. It is a cylinder with a diameter of 25 cm and an equivalent length. Its front face is curved to resist air pressure. The whole unit is mechanically protected against shocks and X-rays.

- Primary screen

It consists of two adjoining parts.

- An X-ray sensitive layer, converting X-ray photons (20 to 120 keV) into light photons (1.5 to 3 keV).

- A photocathode which, under the action of light photons, releases low-energy electrons by photo-electric effect.

- Secondary display

Located at the opposite end of the tube, it collects the accelerated electrons and converts them into photons of light.

- Electrode group

It has two functions:

- The acceleration of the electrons, which acquire an energy corresponding to the potential difference (30 kV).

- Focusing: these electrons are emitted from a surface 22 cm in diameter and projected onto the secondary screen measuring 2 to 3 cm in diameter, maintaining the image of the primary screen.

-The final image is transmitted to a television screen

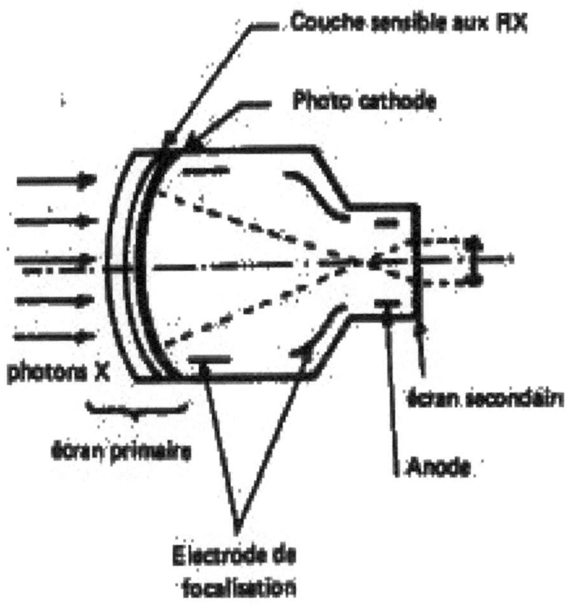

Figure III.14. Luminance amplifier.

- Television camera

It analyzes the dynamic image of the luminance amplifier using an image-analyzer tube, which receives the light image via a fiber-optic system. The scanning tube is a vacuum chamber in which an electron beam emitted by a filament, focused by an electron gun and directed by a deflector winding, scans a photoconductive target, the nature of which varies according to the type of tube. The electron beam scans the target line by line, playing the role of a wandering electrode: it deposits on the target an electric charge that varies over time like the resistance at each point of the target: the output potential difference reproduces the luminance variations of the different points of the image on the secondary screen: it is this signal which, after amplification, gives the video signal that will be digitized (Figure.III.15).

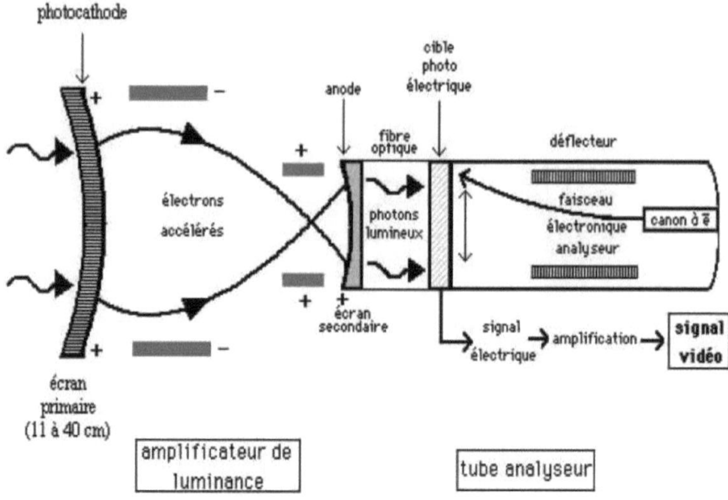

Figure III.15. *Television camera*

VIII.2.2. Memory display

Acquisition is always carried out using a conventional radiology chain: generator, X-ray tube, cassette, with or without the use of a grid. The cassette contains a so-called "memory screen", which replaces the traditional film-screen pair and collects a latent image. The printed cassette is then transferred to a reading unit connected to the image digitization processor. After playback, the information contained on the screen is erased to enable it to be used again. These different stages define an image formation cycle [18] (Figure.III.16).

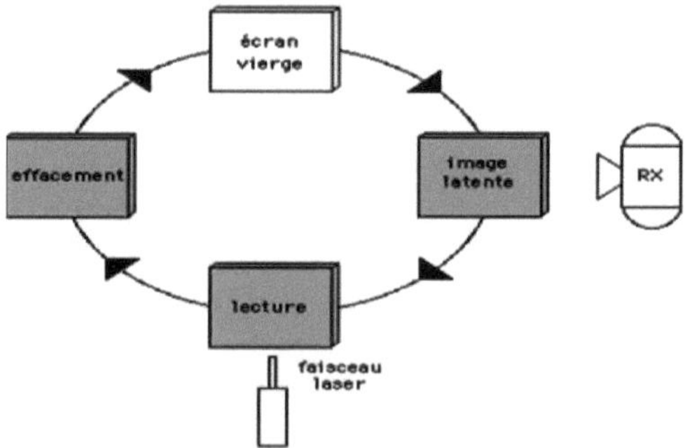

Figure III.16. *Image formation cycle*

The memory screen is made up of four layers:

- Two transparent protective films, one ventral, the other dorsal.

-In between, a luminescent layer of inorganic crystals made of barium fluorohalide doped with divalent europium ions (which acts as an activator).

- A polyethylene support on which the luminescent layer is applied to prevent backscattering.

Images are acquired using photostimulable luminescence in two stages: information gathering, then information reading by photostimulation.

- Information gathering: this takes place on a screen, made up of crystals characterized by their luminescence properties: light emission following excitation phenomena by energy absorption, in this case X-rays. Excitation of the crystal's molecules causes an electron to be projected to a higher energy level; the electron's new energy level is unstable: it will return to its initial level by emitting light, but first passes through an intermediate level called the trap level: this trapping is of variable duration: it is very short in the case of fluorescent emission (instantaneous emission), but longer in the case of phosphorescence (remanent emission) (figure III.17).

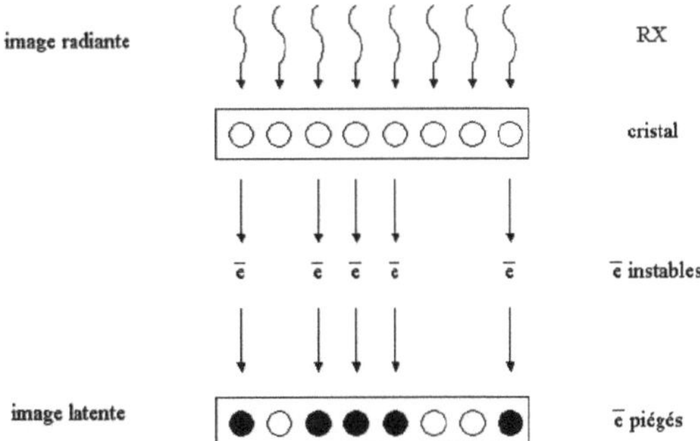

Figure III.17: *Latent image formation.*

- Photostimulation: the second stage is therefore a reading stage: the luminescent emission resulting from the return to the ground state of the trapped electrons requires stimulation of sufficient energy: this is the photostimulation provided by infrared radiation emitted by a laser beam: this scans the screen (reading time: approx. 45 seconds), releases the electrons bound to the halides and triggers light emissions whose intensity will reflect the intensity of the radiant image point by point. These light emissions take place in an emission spectrum that differs from the stimulation spectrum of infrared radiation. Once the laser reading has been taken, any information still present on the screen is erased by exposure to a high-intensity flash of light (such as a sodium lamp), which cleans out the trap levels and makes the screen available again (figure III.18).

- <u>Photomultiplication</u>: the light signal obtained is then transformed into an electrical signal and amplified via a photomultiplier tube. This electrical signal is then digitized.

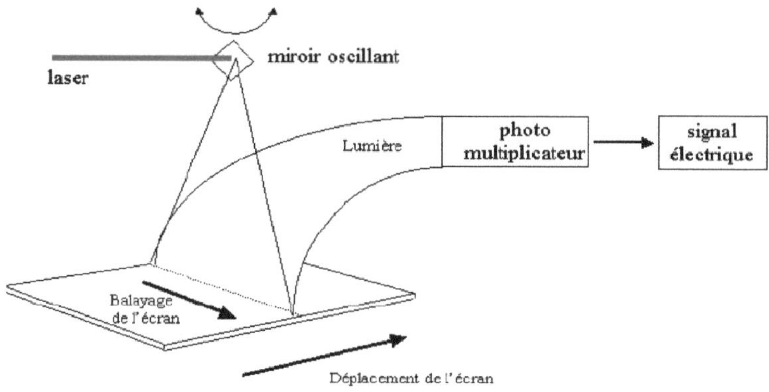

Figure III.18: *Principle of screen reading by photo-stimulation.*

VIII.2.3 Selenium drum

The detector of the radiant image is an amorphous layer of selenium, which is a photo-semiconductor: when exposed to X-rays, it becomes conductive. Exposure to X-rays leads to the formation of electron holes, which partially neutralize the positive charges of the selenium. The residual charges will reflect the radiant image: they will be read by a charge-reading capacitor. The selenium detector is a system dedicated exclusively to thoracic radiography (figure III.19).

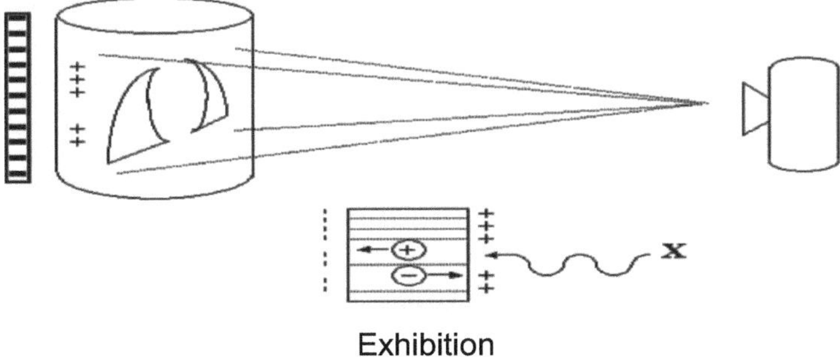

Figure III.19. *Selenium drum*

It consists of a drum 50 cm in diameter and 50 cm high, on which a thin layer of amorphous selenium has been homogeneously vaporized onto an aluminum support. The image is formed in 3 stages:

1. Electric charging: an electric field is created by depositing a positive charge on the surface of the drum while applying a negative charge to the aluminum.
2. Exposure phase: photons from the radiant image are projected onto the surface of the drum, forming electron-hole pairs that are attracted by the positive charges on the surface. The residual charges constitute the latent image.
3. Reading phase: the drum is rotated at high speed, bringing it into contact with an array of charge-reading capacitor detectors. With each rotation, the capacitors (0.2mm) are displaced by 0.1mm and scan the surface of the drum. It is the rotation that enables the horizontal information to be read, and the translation with each revolution that enables the entire height of the drum to be covered. Total reading time is around 10 seconds. The resulting electrical signal is amplified and digitized. The distortion of the latent image due to the curved surface of the drum is corrected by a mathematical algorithm.

VIII.2.4. Planar detector

The device takes the form of a rectangular box with an active surface area ranging from 5 x 5 cm^2 to 60 x 100 cm^2 , and a thickness ranging from 1 to 10 cm. The most common size is that used in human medicine, with 36 x 43 cm^2 (14 x 17 inches^2). These sensors can be divided into two main families:

a. Direct conversion sensors

The sensor is an amorphous selenium-coated substrate onto which a matrix of photodiodes and TFTs (thin-film field-effect transistors) has been deposited.X photons are absorbed by the selenium,   releasing electrical charges. These charges are attracted by an electric field. The electrode of the pixel connected to the transistor is then charged. The charges collected by the matrix are stored before being read and converted into a digital value [19] (figure III.20).

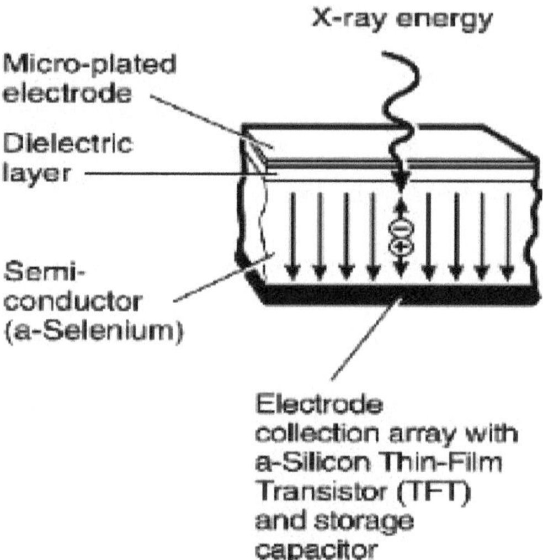

Figure III.20. *Direct conversion of X-rays into electrical signals in contact with a photoconductor.*

b. Indirect conversion sensors

X-rays are transformed into visible photons within the scintillating material (amorphous silicon or selenium technologies). The visible photons are then converted into electrical charges and a digital signal. The sensor is coupled to a photodiode deposited on a TFT layer (figure III.21).

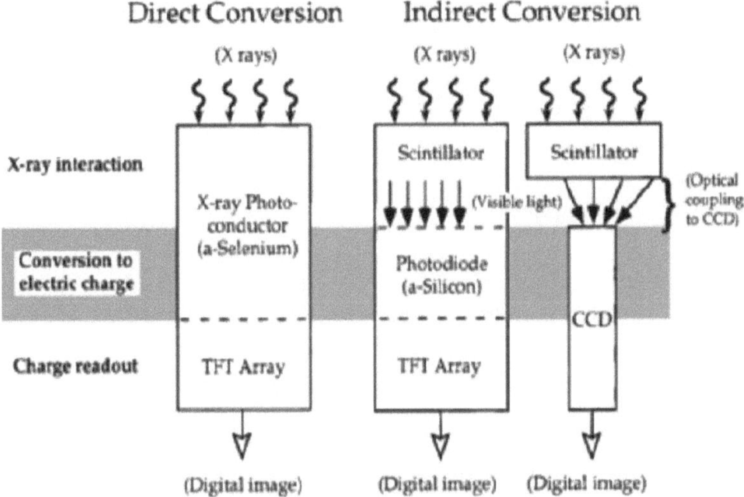

Figure III.21. *Principle of the direct and indirect conversion planar sensor.*

Conclusion

This chapter focuses on a detailed study of one medical imaging modality: conventional and digital radiology. First, the definition of radiology and its principle were presented, followed by a description of the parameters that influence the degradation of the radiological image. Finally, detection systems for conventional and digital radiology were presented.

Exercises

A medical imaging practice has both conventional and digital X-ray equipment for torso, mammography and dental panoramic examinations respectively.

1. What is the benefit of these types of radiological examinations?

2. Show the principle of an X-ray on a diagram

3. Briefly explain the role of each element in the chain?

4. The radiologist performs a mammography examination.

    4.1. Why use digital radiology?

    4.1. What type of anode will be used by the engineer so that the radiologist can carry out a mammography?justify your choice?

5. the X-ray beam undergoes attenuation as it passes through the organ to be studied, and the intensity of the transmitted beam is given by the following law: $I = I_0 \cdot \exp(-kE)$.

Knowing that I_0 is the intensity of the incident beam, k is the absorption coefficient of the organ and E is the thickness through which the beam passes

5.1. Explain the causes (phenomena) of the attenuation of the X-ray beam as it passes through the organ to be studied?

6. On the X-ray shown below (fig.1), a patient's torso is represented. The following information is given:

Main soft tissue components			Main elements present in bones	
Carbon	Hydrogen	Oxygen	Calcium	Phosphorus

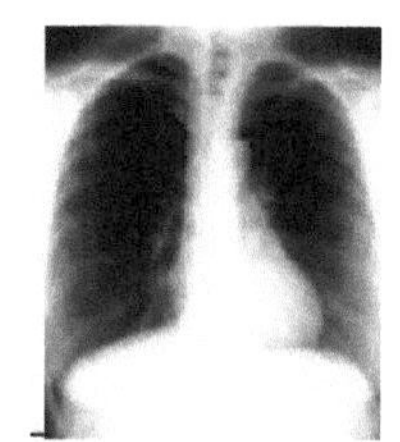

6.1. Explain the principle of the image acquisition system shown in figure.1.

6.2. Interpret the image of the torso obtained by conventional radiography?

6.3. Why can tumors be detected by radiology?

6.4. Explain how the generator voltage should be adjusted to obtain a high-contrast X-ray image (fig.1) ?

6.5. What solution is being considered to increase the contrast of low-contrast soft tissues?

7. The radiologist wishes to carry out a dental panoramic examination.

- What detection system will be used? Explain its operating principle.

8. The doctor asks the patient to have a CT scan. Explain how the engineer should set up the generator and the X-ray tube to obtain the best visual quality slices?

Chapter 4

Classic and modern computed tomography

Introduction

Although X-ray radiography allows us to better observe the image of a part of the human body with a flat surface, it has been limited in three main aspects:

1. The structure of the human body is multi-layered (one organ may be covered by another).
2. It is very difficult to differentiate between tissues within the same organ. Therefore, radiography is never used to treat lesions or tumors.
3. X-rays only give us anatomical images of the human body. It contains no information on the physiology and biology of the living organ.

With a view to solving the problem of the body's multilayered structure, the first scanner was introduced by Godfrey Hounsfield in London in 1971, with the installation of a first "skull" prototype. The invention of X-ray tomography represented one of the first upheavals in medical imaging, and is the basis of the immense progress made in this field. This chapter is divided into two sections. In the first section, we describe the operating principle of a CT scanner. In addition, the various components and slice acquisition systems are described in detail. Next, we describe the phases involved in forming the scenographic image. We then present the different generations of scanners. The second section of the chapter focuses on the modern scanner. Its operating principle and the sensors used in this type of scanner are described. Finally, the parameters of image acquisition and reconstruction are studied.

I.   CT scanner principle

When biological tissue is exposed to X-rays, the latter are attenuated according to an exponential function taking into account photoelectric absorption and Compton scattering. If I_0 is the incident X-ray flux in a heterogeneous medium with attenuation coefficient μ , and I is the flux leaving the tissue, we have the following relationship:

$$I = I0 \exp\text{-}\mu (x) \quad (IV.I)$$

Where: x, thickness of the organ passed through.

The CT scanner is based on the measurement of the different absorption coefficients of tissues crossed by an X-ray beam. Each tissue has its own absorption coefficient, which depends on the density of the tissue and the energy of the beam passing through it. By associating a gray level scale with this coefficient, retro-projection algorithms can be used to obtain a scanner image, corresponding to the image of a cross-section of the body under study [11].

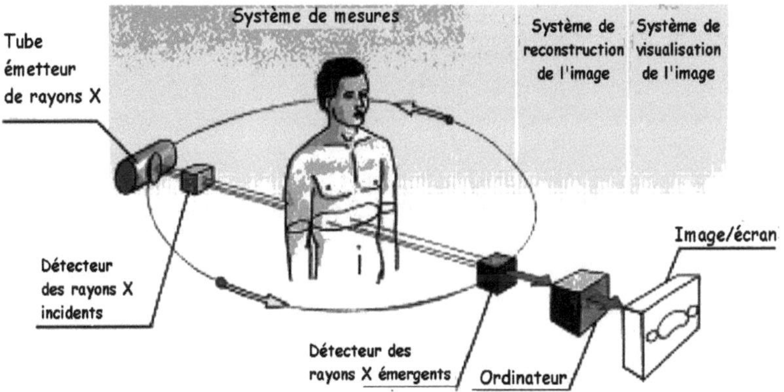

Figure IV.1.*Scanner operation*

II. Scanning chain

A scan chain consists of :
- From tube to X-ray
- Primary and secondary collimation.
- Image acquisition systems,
- A data processing system,
- A visualization system,
- An archiving system.

In this section, we present the different elements of a scan chain (Figure.IV.2).

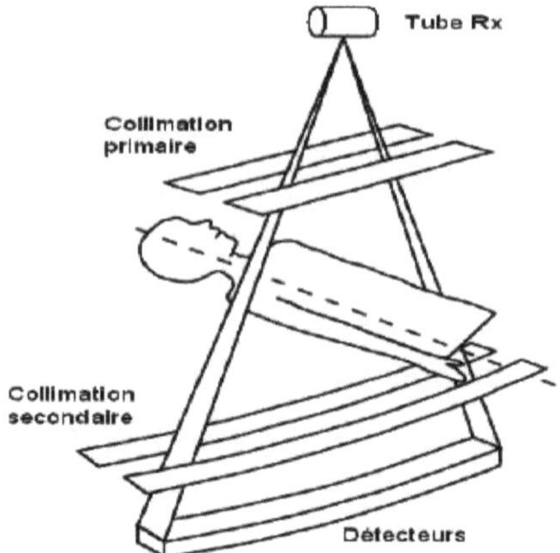

Figure IV.2: *Scanning chain.*

II.1 X-ray generator

The generator delivers high DC voltage (80 to 140 kV) and constant milliamperage (10 to 500 mA). It has a total available power of 50 to 60 kW. It is usually placed in the stand.

II.2 X-ray tube

Modern scanners operate in spiral mode (multi-slice), with extremely rapid acquisition. Tubes must be extremely high-performance. They must be capable of

- Absorb high thermal stresses, hence the need for a high heat capacity (expressed in UC heat units). The most efficient tubes in use today have heat capacities of the order of 5.0 to 7.0 MUC (MUC: Million Heat Units; one Heat Unit = the energy required to raise the temperature of one gram of water by one degree).
- They are rotary anode, with continuous emission.
- They also have to withstand the mechanical stresses of centrifugal force on the latest-generation stands, which rotate at a speed of 0.5 seconds per 360°.

- Another important feature is spatial resolution, which, under certain acquisition conditions, will be limited by the size of the focus (the area where electrons are bombarded onto the anode): this calls for the design of multi-focus tubes (smaller for acquisition in high spatial resolution mode, and larger for acquisition in high contrast resolution mode).

II.3. filter

The filter delimits low-energy X-rays.

II.4 Primary and secondary collimation

- **he primary collimation** is located downstream of the filter. It calibrates the X-ray beam according to the desired cut thickness.
- **Secondary collimation** is placed before the detector. It must be perfectly aligned with the focus and primary collimation. It limits the radiation scattered by the patient.

III. Detection systems

Detectors are used to transform X-ray photons into an electrical signal, and two types can be distinguished:

III.1 Xenon ionization chambers

Xenon's properties form the basis of the detector. Under the action of the rays, the electrons are excited and produce an electric current. It is this signal that is recovered, signals proportional to the attenuation of the body through which they pass [20].

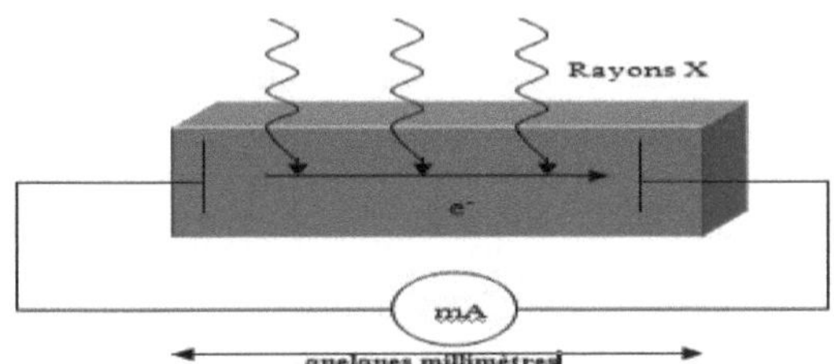

Figure IV.3: *Xenon detector*

III.2 Solid state detector

Today, all scanners are equipped with solid-state detectors. They are sometimes incorrectly referred to as semiconductors. These detectors maximize detection efficiency and therefore contrast resolution per dose delivered to the patient.

This detector consists of crystals placed in an ionization chamber. These crystals receive X-rays, converting them into light energy that is proportional to the intensity of the beam received. A photodiode recovers this light intensity and converts it into electrical signals (figure IV.4).

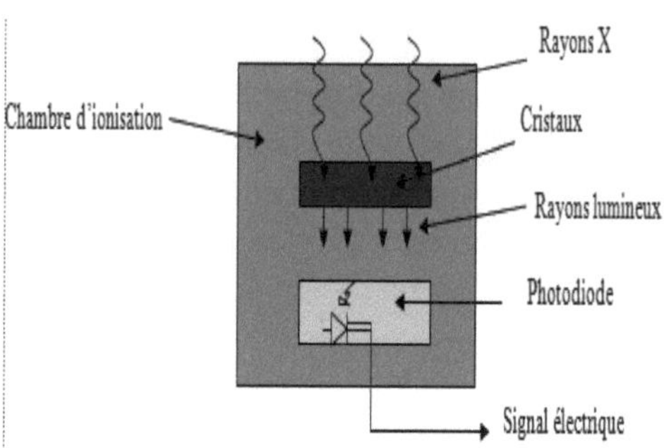

Figure IV.4. *Solid state detector*

The detector consists of one or more strips arranged in a fan-like pattern. Each bar provides the information required to reconstruct a section. For example, a scanner with n strips can simultaneously acquire n slices by rotation. Each bar contains several hundred sensors.

III.3 Stand

The stand (housing X-ray tube, detector and generator) with a tunnel (through which the patient can pass) perpendicular to the table axis; it is fixed, but can be tilted +/- 25° from the vertical.

The scanner stand consists of two main parts: the stator and the rotor.

    a. Stator

Is the fixed part. It comprises the following elements:

- the tunnel (usually 70 cm in diameter)
- mechanical control elements for various stand movements

    b. Rotor

Is the moving part. It contains :

- high-voltage generator (for X-ray production)
- X-ray tube and cooling circuits

- the detection system and associated electronics, some high-speed processors and the data transmission system.

Rotor speeds are generally of the order of a second for 360° rotation. The current trend is to increase rotation speed. Most manufacturers offer devices that complete a full revolution in around 0.5 sec. This is useful for functional examinations (perfusion) and for imaging fast-moving organs (heart). Increasing rotation speed must necessarily be accompanied by an increase in instantaneous X-ray power, to avoid degrading image quality.

IV. Forming tomographic images

There are 3 slices for tomographic image acquisition (figure IV.5):

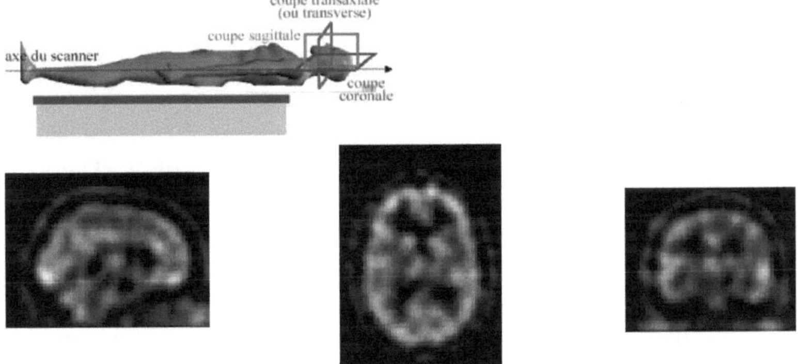

Figure IV.5. *Tomographic sections*

The principle is based on measuring the attenuation of an X-ray beam passing through a segment of the body as it rotates around the patient. X-ray beams passing through an object undergo attenuation by absorption, which depends on the atomic composition of the tissue and the energy of the incident X-rays (figure IV.7). Multiple attenuation profiles are obtained at different rotation angles spread over 360° (figure IV.9 and 10). They are sampled and digitized. The data are back-projected onto a reconstruction matrix and transformed into an analog image. Each pixel is assigned a gray level corresponding to its absorption coefficient. By moving the patient horizontally, it is possible to obtain as many slices as required for diagnosis. The summation of all the density profiles obtained for these different angular values as a function of the attenuation coefficients is called a sinogram [21] (Figure.IV.6).

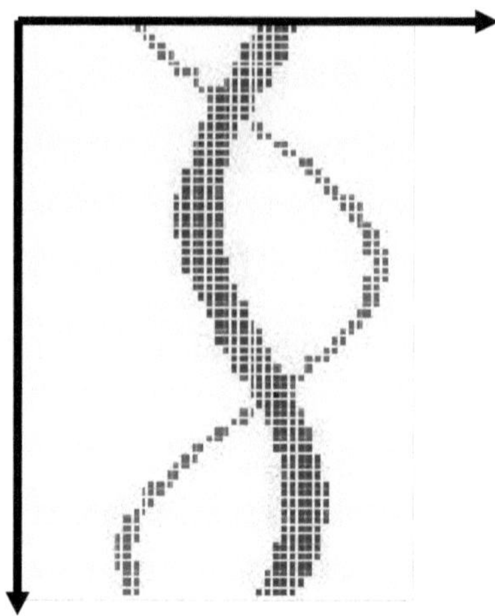

Figure IV.6. *Sinogram*

IV.1 Mitigation

An X-ray beam passing through a homogeneous object of thickness x undergoes attenuation as a function of the object's electron density (Figure IV 7). Attenuation is defined by the relation :

$$\text{Log } I_o/I = \mu x \text{ (IV.II)}$$

Where: I_o: incident beam intensity; I: emergent intensity; μ: attenuation coefficient of the crossed object; x: object thickness.

The beam encounters structures of different density and thickness. Attenuation therefore depends on several unknowns $\mu_1 x_1$, $\mu_2 x_2,...\mu_n x_n$.

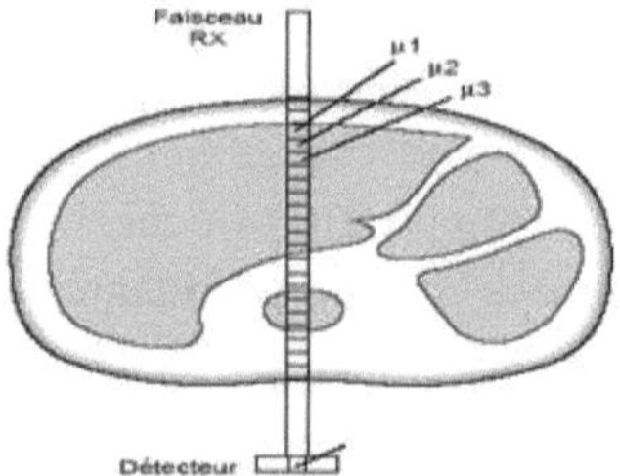

Figure IV.7. *Beam attenuation a RX*

IV.2 Projection

The detector transforms the X-ray photons into an electrical signal (figure IV.8). This signal is directly proportional to the intensity of the X-ray beam. The attenuation profile or projection corresponds to the set of electrical signals provided by all the detectors for a given angle of rotation (figure IV.9). A rotational movement around the long axis of the object to be examined records a series of attenuation profiles resulting from the crossing of the same section at different angles of rotation (figure IV.10).

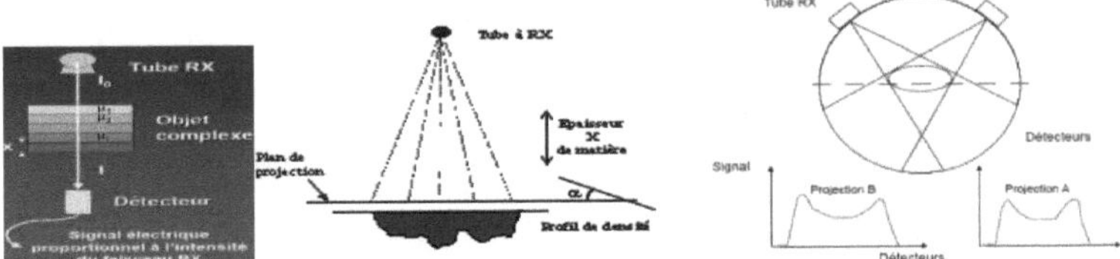

Figure IV.8. Beam attenuation Figure IV.9. Density profile figure IV.10. Multiple profiles

IV.3 Back-projection

With *n* projections obtained from different angles, it is possible to reconstruct an image of the section plane under study. These projections are then back-projected onto a reconstruction matrix. Each attenuation profile is projected at the same angle as during acquisition.

From the attenuation values measured by each detector, the computer calculates the density of each pixel in the matrix. These complex calculations are based on a simple principle: knowing the sum of the numbers in a matrix along all its axes (rows, columns and diagonals), we can deduce all the numbers contained in the matrix.

Example:

$P_1 (1) = a + f + k + p + u = 5$
$P_1 (2) = b + g + l + q + v = 5$
$P_1 (3) = c + h + m + r + w = 20$

. . . .

$P_3 (1) = a + b + c + d + e = 0$
$P_3 (2) = f + g + h + i + j = 25$
$P_3 (3) = k + l + m + n + o = 5$

. . . .

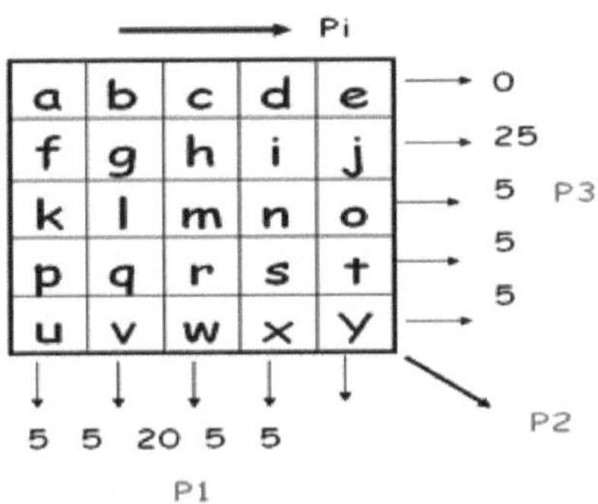

25 equations with 25 unknowns
*For a 128*128 image: 16384 equations*

These mathematical operations require powerful computing resources that can only be obtained by computers. Early CT scanner prototypes only imaged the brain, using a series of sensors arranged in an arc around the head. To produce a single image on these devices, it took two and a half hours to calculate a single tomographic slice from this signal. The first CT images of the brain clearly showed the cavities of the cerebrospinal fluid-filled ventricles. Subsequent machines were able to reconstruct images of all parts of the human body. The Radon transform method (1917) is more commonly used to improve calculation time and image quality of the reconstructed object, and to bring it closer to the initial model.

IV.4. From matrix to image

A matrix is an array of n rows and m columns defining a number of elementary squares or pixels. Current matrices are usually 512*512 . Each pixel in the reconstruction matrix has a corresponding attenuation or density value. Depending on its density, each pixel is represented on the image by a certain gray-scale value. The density coefficients of the various tissues are expressed in Hounsfield units (HU).

- Hounsfield scale

The range varies from -1000 to +1000. With the choice of a value of zero for water, -1000 for air and +1000 for bone (figure.IV.11). The mathematical formula that relates the density coefficient $\mu(x)$ of a given body (x) in Hounsfield units (HU) is given by :

$$\text{Unit (HS)} = \frac{\mu - \mu_{eau}}{\mu_{eau}} * 1000 \qquad\qquad \text{(IV.II)}$$

Hounsfield defined a density scale where: Water = 0 HU; Air = - 1000 HU; Bone = + 1000 HU; Fat = - 50; Brain = +30, +40; Coagulated blood = +80.

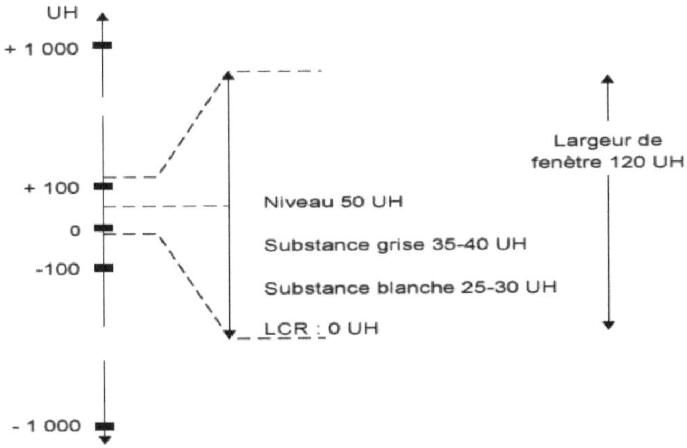

Figure .V.11. *Hounsfield scale.*

Since the human eye can only distinguish 16 levels of gray, all 2,000 density levels cannot be seen simultaneously on the screen, hence the importance of choosing the study window. The window corresponds to the densities that will actually be translated into gray levels on the screen. Any pixel with a value greater than the upper limit of the window is displayed as white, and any pixel with a value less than the lower limit of the window is displayed as black. Two parameters define the useful density window.

1. level: central value of displayed densities (the middle of the Hounsfield unit interval displayed).

2. window width: determines the number of density levels (chosen density interval, in which all the NGs visible to the eye on the screen will be represented).

- By increasing the window, the image is enriched with gray levels, but the contrast between image structures decreases. Decreasing the window increases contrast.

- When the study window is opened as wide as possible, the bone appears white, the air black and all other structures uniformly grey, the image obtained is that of a mediocre conventional tomography.

Depending on the level and width of the window in the Hounsfield absorption scale, the following will be objectified: soft tissue (muscle, heart, liver....), calcium structures (bone) enabling precise study of brain densities) (figure IV.12).

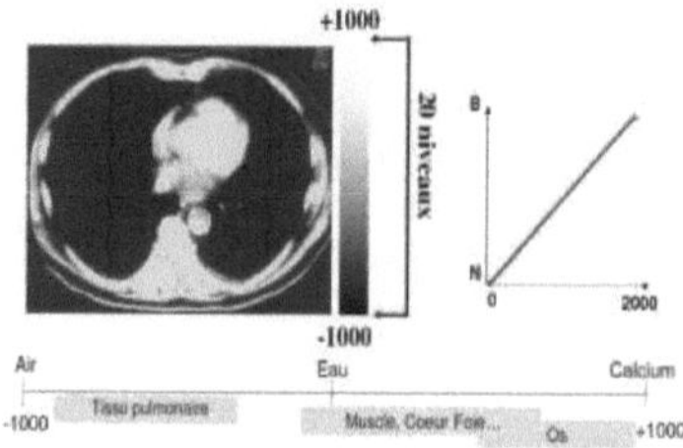
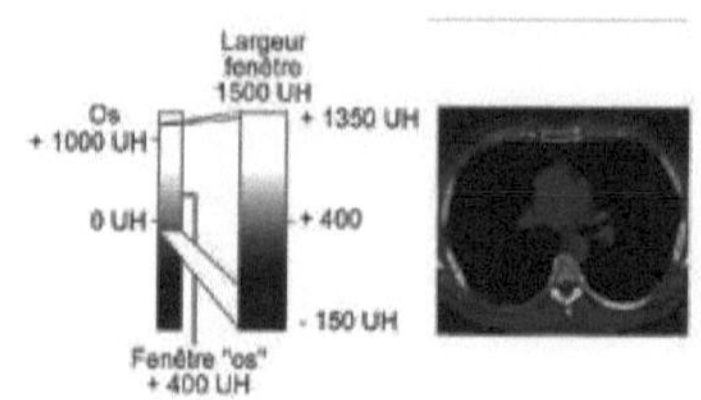

Total window Os window

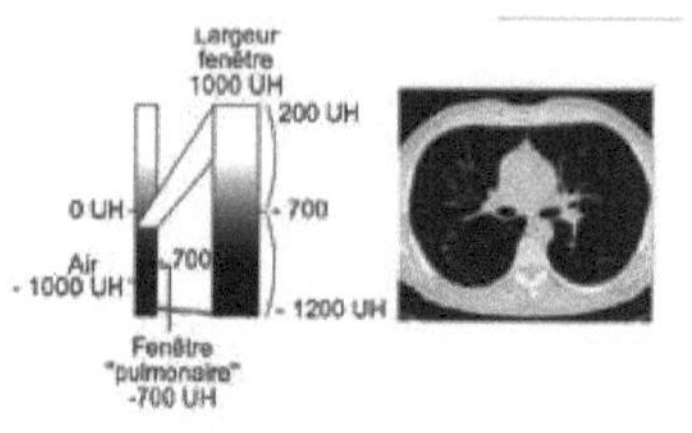
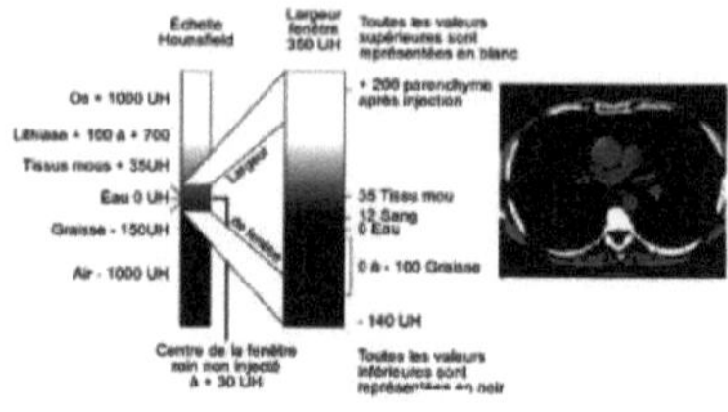

Window air window soft fabric

Figure IV.12.*Density window for different fabrics*

- for soft tissue N= +35 L= +350
- for bone: N = +400 L= + 1500
- for lungs: N= - 700 L= 1000

V. Scanner generation

Since 1976, scanners have benefited from the evolution of information technology. At present, the big industrial firms manufacturing scanners are: philips, siemens, and general electric. There are four generations of classic scanners:

V.1. 1ᵉʳᵉ generation scanner

The 1st generation of scanners combined translation and rotation of the tube to perform a cut (using a single detector) (Figure IV.13). After longitudinal scanning (translation), the assembly is rotated by a small angle around the center of the section under examination (rotation), and a new scan is performed.

During each translation, several hundred measurements are taken to produce a profile of the cross-section at the angle of incidence in question.

-Once the tube-detector pair has rotated through 360° (and a cut has been obtained), the table advances by a chosen increment, and a new cut can be acquired. This is why we speak of incremental mode (slice-by-slice acquisition).

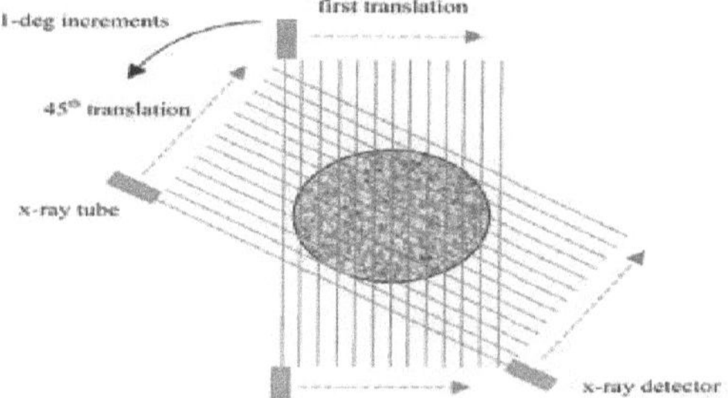

Figure IV.13.*1ᵉʳᵉ scanner generation s*

V.2. 2ᵉᵐᵉ generation scanner

It is still based on the principle of translation-rotation, but the number of detectors is increased (two detectors) (figure IV.14), enabling the acquisition of two simultaneous slices in several minutes, and the beam geometry is modified (aperture angle 10° to 20°). Having several detectors instead of just one increases the rotation increment. Once tube a has rotated 360° around the patient for a given table position z, the table moves forward by one increment and a new rotation of the tube-detector system can take place. We are therefore still in an incremental mode. The handicap of the 2ᵉᵐᵉ generation is that it has a very long acquisition time (several minutes) and is used more for imaging parts of the body than the head.

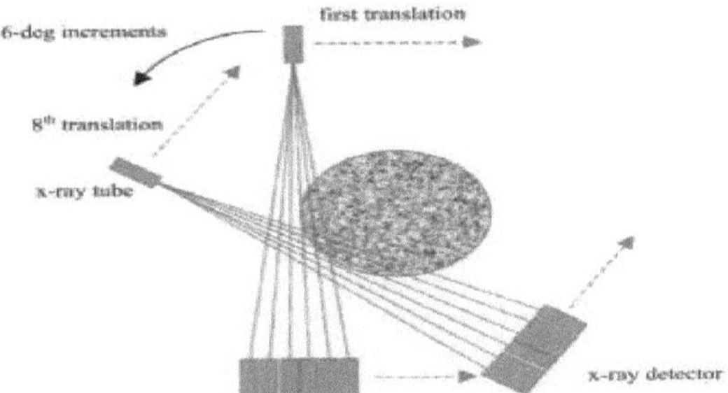

Figure IV.14. *2ᵉᵐᵉ Scanner generation*

V.3. 3 ʳᵈ generation scanner

This is a single-rotation system (rotation-rotation geometry). The tube and detectors rotate at the same time around the patient (Figure IV.15). To eliminate translational movement, a ring of detectors (500 to 1000) is deployed in a circular arc, and the X-ray beam aperture angle is large enough to cover the entire cross-section of the patient, even at the widest point. Once the tube-detector pair has rotated 360° around the patient for a given table position z, the table is advanced by one increment and a further rotation of the tube-detector system can take place. By eliminating the translation step, time resolution has been improved.

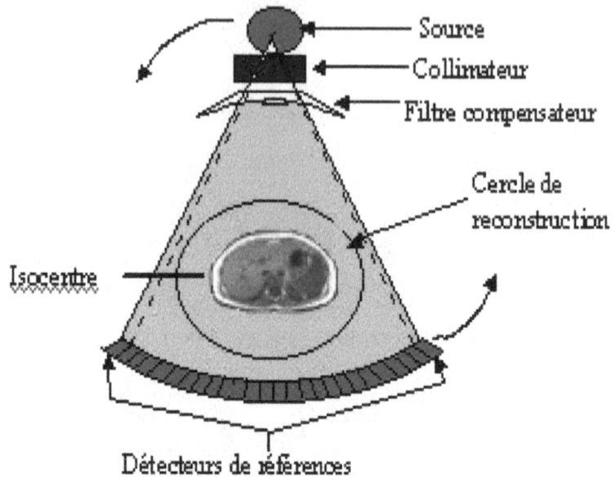

Figure IV.15.*3ᵉᵐᵉ scanner generation*

V.4. Scanner 4ᵉᵐᵉ generation

This is a single-rotation system (stationary-rotation geometry) (Figure IV.16). Thousands of detectors form a complete ring around the ring; only the X-ray tube rotates around the object under examination, and is closer to the object than the detectors as it rotates. This generation is known as a short-geometry scanner, as the beam aperture is much wider to cover the entire object under examination. The number of profiles obtained is limited by the number of detectors surrounding the patient [22]. Because the tube is closer to the object, spatial resolution is relatively degraded. 2,000 to 4,800 detectors are needed for a scanner with good performance.

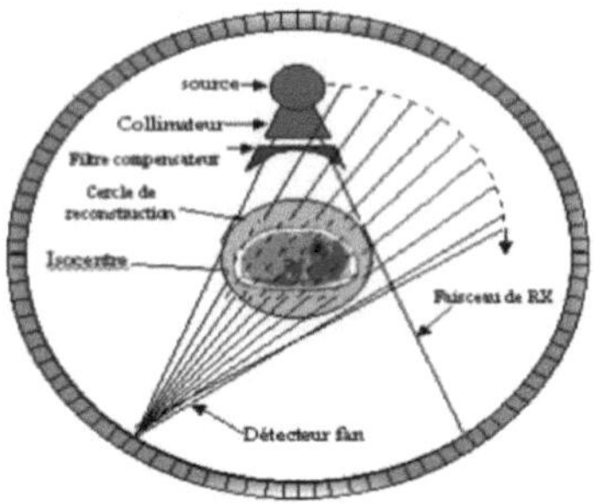

Figure IV.16. *Scanners 4ᵉᵐᵉ Generation*

VI. Modern scanners

Until 1989, only the sequential acquisition mode was used. A cut is acquired at each 360° rotation, in a fixed cutting plane, then the table moves forward to make the next cut. This procedure is repeated cut after cut. In 1989, continuous rotation was introduced, followed by spiral or helical acquisition. Continuous rotation in sequential mode saves considerable time between each cut, avoiding the need to brake and restart the stand. It is still used today for certain indications. But it is helical acquisition that will open up new perspectives in CT.

VI.1. principle of helical scanning

The principle is based on continuous rotation of the tube around the bed, with simultaneous movement of the table as the X-ray beam is scanned. The X-ray beam describes a helix-like geometric pattern around the patient (figure IV.17). At present, most machines use continuous rotation. The speed of rotation on the most recent scanners has been considerably increased, reaching 360° in 0.4 seconds [23].

The result of the helical sequence is a continuous volume of digital data, the length of which corresponds to the movement of the examination bed during acquisition. Sections can be reconstructed at any point in the volume.

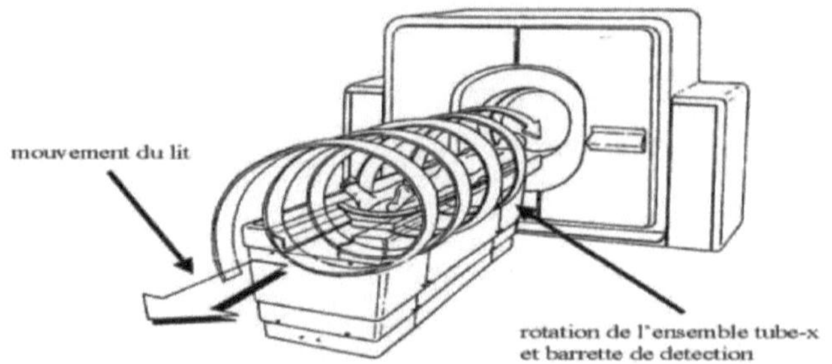

Figure IV.17. *Helical Scanner*

VI.1.1. Single-slice scanner

The single-slice scanner features a single ring of detectors in the Z axis. Between 500 and 900 elements are arranged in the X axis. A single slice is acquired per rotation (figure IV.18).

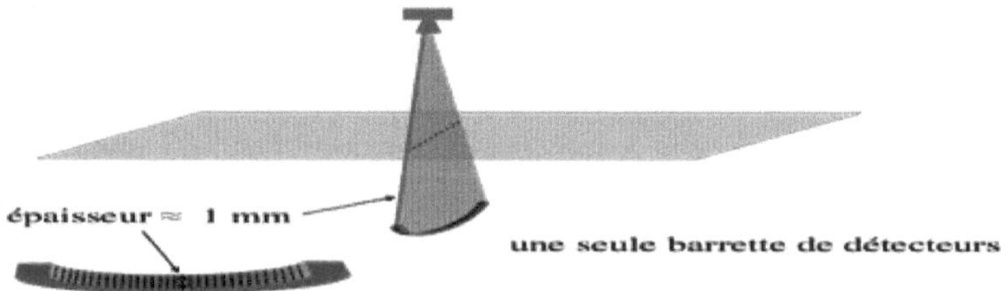

Figure IV.18. Single-slice scanner

VI.1.2. Multi-slice scanner

The evolution of the detection system towards the multi-cut scanner (figure IV.19) is characterized by the subdivision of the detector ring in the Z axis into two to 34 rings made up of detectors of varying number and thickness, depending on the technological solutions proposed by the manufacturers.

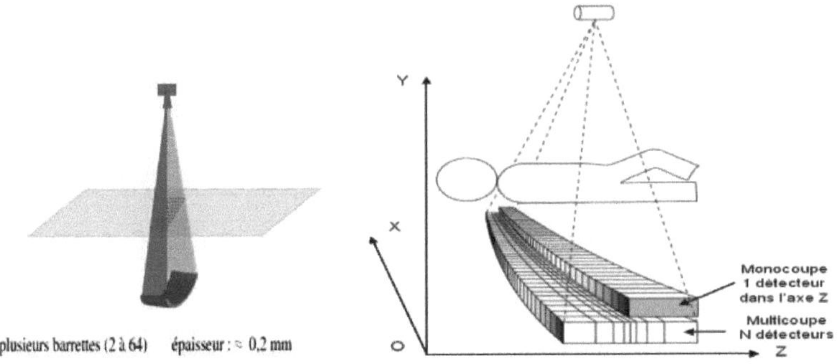

Figure IV.19. *Comparison of the detection system in single-slice and multi-slice scanners. The Oz axis is the patient's axis.*

VI.2 Detector arrangement

The arrangement of detectors in the Z axis varies according to the manufacturer and the number of simultaneous cuts possible (Figure IV.20). Three types of detectors can be distinguished:

VI.2.1. Symmetrical

All detectors have the same width. They can acquire from 2 to 8 slices simultaneously.

VI.2.2. Asymmetrical

The width of the detectors increases as they move away from the perpendicular to the axis of rotation. The use of wider peripheral detectors compensates for the cone effect.

VI.2.3. Hybrids

The detectors are of two different widths. At present, they allow from 2 to 16 simultaneous cuts to be obtained. ballast composed of 34 detectors, four 0.5 mm central detectors and 15 1 mm detectors on either side , creating a 32 mm wide ring. As with matrix detectors, it is the individual or grouped activation of the detectors that produces the desired cut thickness. This is the only detector capable of obtaining 4 simultaneous sub-centimeter cuts (0.5 mm).

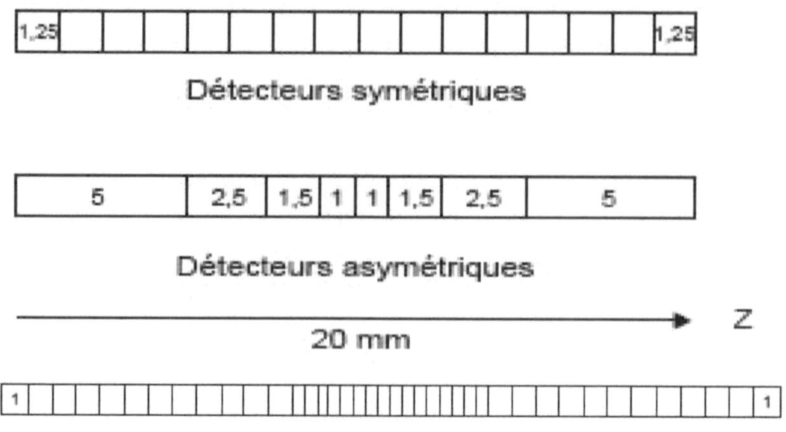

Figure IV.20. *The three types of detectors in multi-slice scanners.*

Depending on the technological options offered by manufacturers, the number and width of detectors govern :
- Minimum cut thickness available (up to 0.5 mm).
- Number of cuts made with minimum thickness (2 to 4).
- Range of cut thicknesses available (from 0.5 to 10 mm) (figure IV.21).
- Maximum thickness of volume covered by rotation (currently 20 to 32 mm).

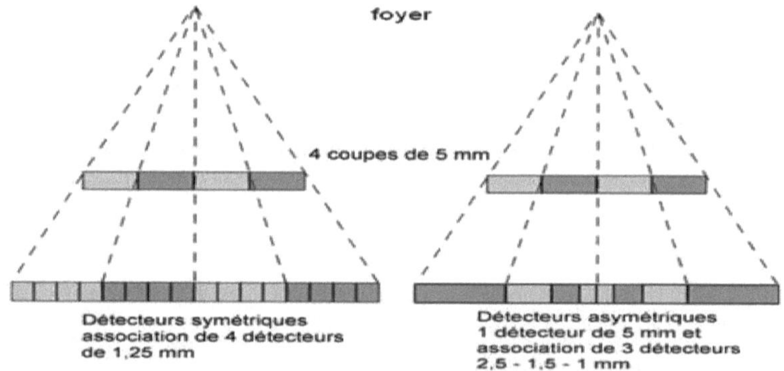

Figure IV.21. *5 mm cross-section using a combination of symmetrical and asymmetrical detectors*

- Principle of the cone effect

The main factor limiting the number of simultaneous slices per rotation is the cone artifact. On multi-slice scanners, the projection of the X-ray beam in the Z axis represents a cone. The central rows of detectors are reached perpendicularly to the axis of rotation, while the outermost rows are reached obliquely by the X-rays. This obliquity degrades image quality at the periphery. When a peripheral detector is activated in isolation, the width of the volume traversed by the X-ray beam becomes greater than the width of the detector. This obliquity also reduces the efficiency of the peripheral detectors. If several detectors are combined, or if the peripheral detector is wider, the width of the volume traversed is close to the cut thickness (figure IV.22).

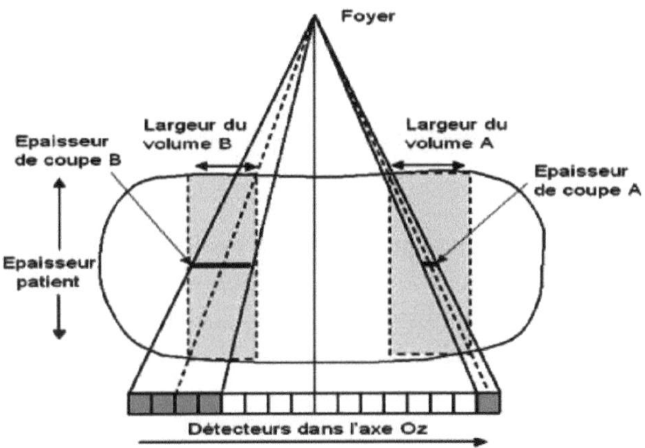

Figure IV.22. *Cone effect.*

VI.3 System architecture according to number of cuts

Today's scanners simultaneously use 4 real or combined crowns to acquire 4 simultaneous slices per rotation.

VI.3.1.Systems 2 cuts

This is the first generation of multi-slice scanners. Two detector rings of identical size in the Z axis are combined, enabling simultaneous acquisition of two slices whose thickness depends on primary and secondary collimation.

VI.3.2.4-cut systems

They comprise four rings of varying thickness. Two types of detector arrangement are available: symmetrical and asymmetrical.

    a. Symmetrical detectors: these comprise 16 1.25 mm wide detectors in the Z axis. The desired cut thickness is obtained by activating the detectors (1.25 mm wide) in groups of one, two, three or four detectors, to obtain 4 cuts of 1.25 mm, 2.5 mm, 3.75 mm or 5 mm (figure IV 23). Only the acquisition of 5 mm slices uses all detectors in the z axis.

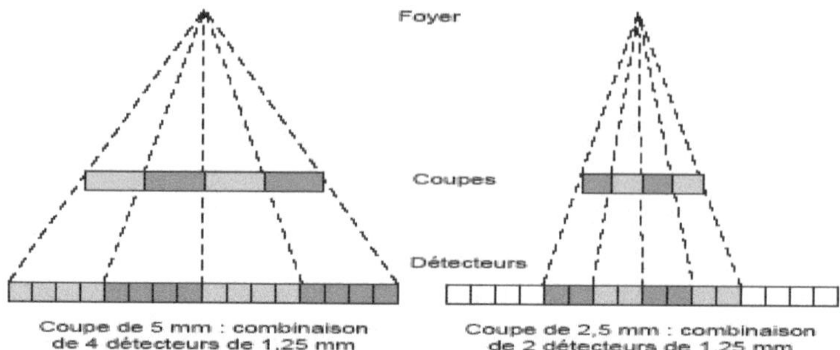

Figure IV.23. *Symmetrical detectors: combination of detectors depending on the desired cutting thickness.*

b. Asymmetrical detectors: these are made up of 8 detectors of increasing width, from 1 to 5mm, and can obtain 2 cuts of 0.5mm or 4 cuts of 1 to 5mm; it is the adjustment of the secondary collimation that determines the cut thickness (figure IV. 24).

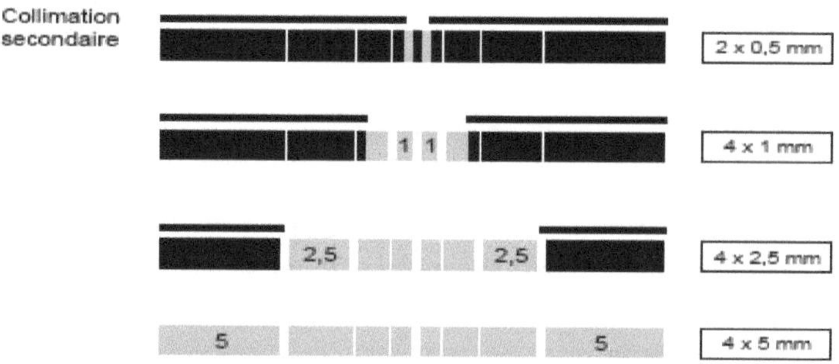

Figure IV.24. *Asymmetrical detectors: combining detectors and adjusting secondary collimation according to the desired cutting thickness.*

VII. Image acquisition and reconstruction

VII.1. Acquisition parameters

VII.1.1. Primary collimation and nominal thickness

It is defined by the collimation width of the X-ray beam at the tube outlet. It determines the nominal cut thickness in single-slice acquisition. It can vary from 1 to 10 mm. In multi-slice scanners, a distinction must be made between nominal thickness and collimation (nominal thickness * number of slices per revolution). Collimation varies according to the number and thickness of cuts available. Current primary collimation values range from 1 mm for 2 slices of 0.5 mm to 32 mm for 4 slices of 8 mm.

VII.1.2. Rotation time

For several years now, single-slice helical scanners have been able to achieve 360° acquisition times of 0.75 to 0.8 seconds. The rotation time is 0.5 seconds for 360° on the most recent multi-slice machines, and all examinations can benefit from this rotation speed. It is sometimes useful to increase this rotation time to benefit from more measurements (projections) per rotation and improve image quality (for example, when studying the shoulder girdle).

VII.1.3. Pitch

Pitch is defined as the ratio between the pitch of the helix (distance covered by the table during a 360° rotation of the tube) and the collimation of the X-ray beam.

Example: during a pitch 1 acquisition, the examination table is displaced by the collimation thickness).

- Single-cut acquisition

Collimation corresponds to the nominal cutting thickness (Figure IV.25).

- Multi-slice acquisition

This is no longer the case in multi-slice acquisition, where collimation corresponds to 4 times the nominal slice thickness, or more precisely 4 times the width of a detector *(scanner has four bars and its table movement is four times faster than a scanner table with a bar pitch of 1)*. The value of the pitch is therefore no longer the same from one manufacturer to another, depending on whether the pitch is calculated on the basis of collimation (collimation pitch) or on the basis of the nominal acquisition thickness and therefore the width of a detector (detection pitch).

Example: if we choose an acquisition with a nominal thickness of 2.5 mm, i.e. a detector width of 2.5 mm and a collimation of 10 mm, a table displacement of 15 mm per revolution will correspond to a collimation pitch of 1.5 (15/10) and a detection pitch of 6 (15/2.5) (Figure.IV.25). A displacement of 7.5 mm per revolution corresponds to a collimation pitch of (7.5/10) 0.75 and a detection pitch of 3(7.5/2.5) (partial beam overlap) (Figure.IV.26).

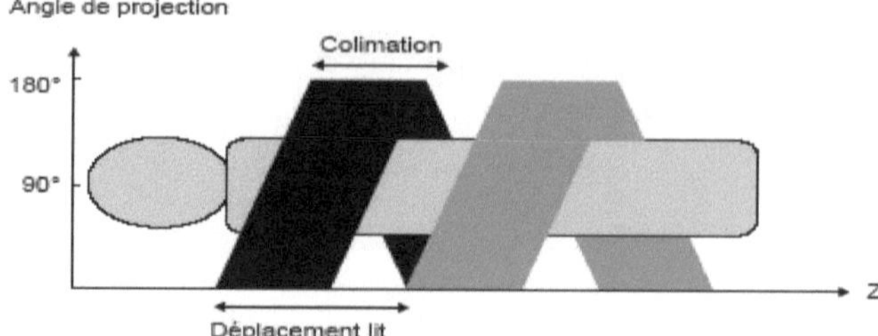

Figure IV.25. *Single-slice scanner: pitch 1.5.*

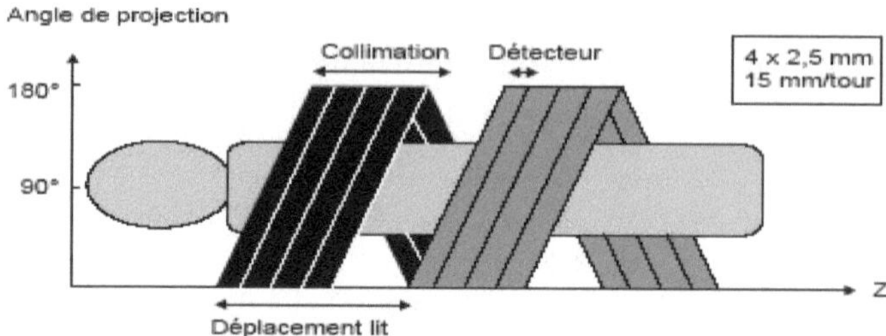

Figure IV.26. *Multislice scanner (4 simultaneous slices) detection pitch of 6 and collimation pitch of 1.5.*

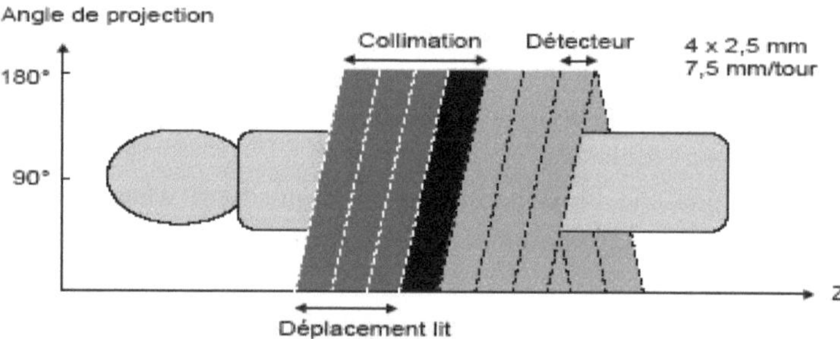

Figure IV.27. *Multi-slice scanner (4 simultaneous slices) detection pitch of 3 and collimation pitch of 0.75. Partial beam overlap from one rotation to the next.*

The choice of collimation pitch better reflects the geometry of the beam around the patient, with overlap from one rotation to the next for pitches below 1. Manufacturers offer collimation pitches ranging from 0.5 to 2. Using pitches lower than 1 exposes the helices to partial overlap.

VII.2.Reconstruction parameters

VII.2.1. Reconstruction filter

The attenuation profiles collected by the detectors are Fourier-transformed into a frequency range before the back-projection stage. The frequency spectra also undergo a filtering function. The selection of high frequencies by "hard" or spatial filters favors representation of the anatomical limits of structures, while making image noise more visible.

Conversely, the elimination of high frequencies by "soft" or density filters attenuates noise and the visibility of contours, enabling better discrimination of structures with low density differences.

-These filters optimize the reconstructed image according to the structure being studied. Soft" filters are suitable for low-contrast structures, and hard filters for structures with naturally high contrast, such as bone and lung.

VII.2.2. Reconstruction matrix

The reconstruction matrix is usually 512x512. On some machines, it can go up to 1024 x1024 in high-resolution mode.

VII.2.3. Interpolation algorithms

In helical scanning, the raw data (digitized projections) cannot be used directly (unlike in sequential mode) due to the continuous movement of the patient during acquisition. If images are reconstructed directly from this data, image quality will be impaired by motion artifacts. It is therefore essential to calculate plane raw data from volume data. This calculation is performed using interpolation algorithms.

The data projection of a helix can be represented as an oblique line. Each point on the line represents a projection (Figure IV.28), indexed to the Oz axis due to the bed displacement, and corresponding to a precise angle of rotation.

If we consider a reconstruction plane at a precise position in the Oz axis, only one point on the helix crosses the reconstruction plane: only one projection is actually measured. All other projections of the 0° to 360° cutting plane must be interpolated.

- In single-slice scanners: Interpolation algorithms are linear and sometimes accessible to the operator, who can choose between two of the most frequently used interpolation algorithms:

- the 360° linear algorithm: this interpolates data measured at two identical angular positions before and after the position of the reconstruction plane. It therefore uses data from two 360° rotations (Figure IV.28).

- the 180° linear algorithm: this is similar to the 360° linear algorithm, but uses only data acquired during a 360° rotation. Missing projections are considered similar to those measured with the symmetrical angle. For example, data obtained at 270 (90° + 180°) are similar to those collected at 90° (figure IV.29).

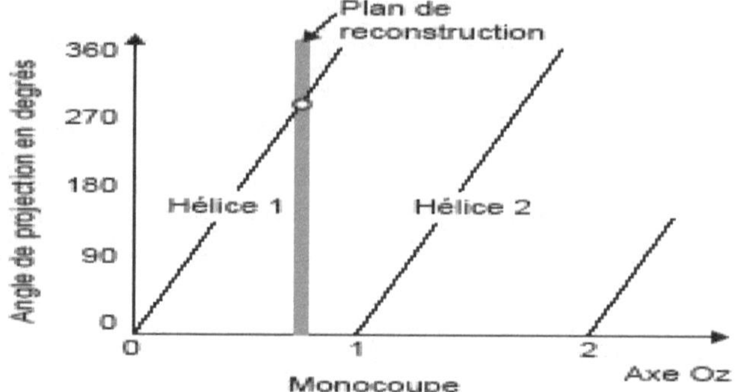

Figure IV.28. *Data projection of a helix in a single-cut helical scanner*

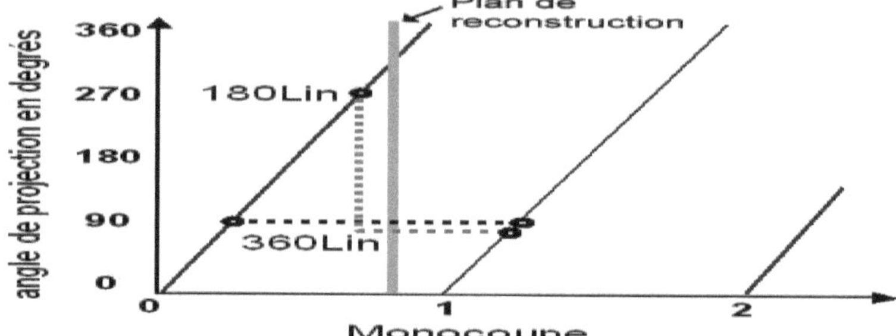

Figure IV.29.*180° and 360° linear reconstruction algorithms for single-slice scanners.*

- Multi-cut scanner

With multi-slice scanners, 4 measurements can be collected at each angular position by 360° rotation. Interpolation is no longer limited to two measurements as with single-slice scanners, but can be performed from several points. There are certain pitches where some of the data from two successive helices overlap and are redundant. These pitches are unfavorable for optimal data interpolation. This explains why some machines do not offer all pitch values (figure IV.30).

- *Pitch<1: two overlapping propellers, so Pitch must be >1 to avoid problems.*

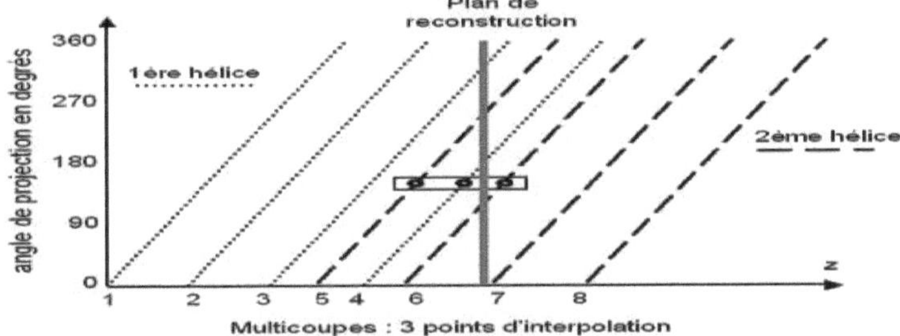

Figure IV.30. *Linear reconstruction algorithm for multi-slice CT scanners*

VIII. Advantages of multi-bar scanners

Multi-slice scanners offer three advantages over single-slice scanners: increased acquisition speed, a clear improvement in image quality, and variable slice thickness.

VIII.1 Acquisition speed

The very high acquisition speeds of these scanners mean shorter acquisition times than with a single-barrier scanner, and the thermal load on the tube is reduced accordingly. This speed of acquisition offers clear advantages:

- improves exploration of fragile patients
- makes it easier to obtain shorter apneas during the acquisition of mobile structures
- reduces the amount of contrast medium injected
- makes it easier to isolate the vascular phases of different organs.

VIII.2 Longitudinal spatial resolution

The improvement in longitudinal spatial resolution is due to the possibility of using fine collimation with a satisfactory section profile, even when the volume covered is large. The use of ultrathin sections enables us to approach isotropic acquisition, thus improving exploration of rock or small bone structures. Finally, it is now possible to explore very large segments without sacrificing image quality, enabling angio-scans of the lower limbs and aorto-iliac exploration to be carried out in a single step.

VIII.3 Variable cutting thickness

Several cut thicknesses are available from a single acquisition. There is a clear advantage in being able to modify the cut thickness after the fact.

IX.   Scanner limitations

1. Direct vertical cuts impossible, but this limitation disappears with the possibility of reconstructing cuts in different planes with ever greater precision.

2. In many cases, it is necessary to inject an iodinated contrast medium to improve contrast, particularly of the various parenchyma and vessels.

3. Some artifacts may degrade the image: these are less annoying than in MRI and rarely render exploration uninformative.

Conclusion

This chapter is devoted to the study of another medical imaging technique: conventional and helical CT. On the one hand, we have presented the principle of CT scanning and the various elements in the scanning chain. On the other hand, image acquisition systems in conventional and modern CT have been detailed, and we have ended this chapter with a description of **CT** image reconstruction methods.

Exercises

Exercise 1

The energy of a photon is E_{ph} = 50 keV.

    1. Determine the wavelength of this photon.

    2. What type of photon is it, and why?

    3. What are the main characteristics of this type of radiation?

Knowing that: 1 eV = 1.6 10-19 J, Planck's constant (h)= h = 6.62 10-34 J.s. And air speed c= 3.00 108 m.s-1

4. Give a diagram of the scan chain and briefly explain the role of each component?

5. What are the characteristics of the X-ray tube used in CT scanning?

6. What do Figures 1 and 2 represent?

7. What do the pixel values in Figure 2 mean?

8. Explain how you could visualize the lungs (fig.3) from figures 1 and 2?

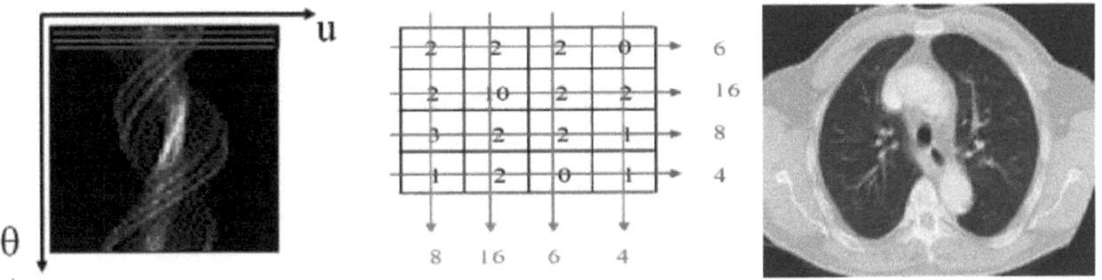

Fig. 1 Fig.2 Fig 3

9. The doctor plans to acquire 4 contiguous sections of the brain to reconstruct the volume.

9.1. What type of scanner is used? Explain its operating principle?

9.2. To obtain these cross-sections, the engineer uses asymmetrical detectors.

9.2.1 What is the architecture of this type of detector and why is it useful?

9.2.2. Propose the architecture of a system capable of acquiring 4 slices of 2.5 mm.

9.2.3. Calculate the parameters that the manipulator must adjust to obtain the 4 cuts, given that the table moves 10 mm per revolution.

Exercise 2

In a medical imaging center, a doctor asks the patient to undergo a helical CT scan of the cervical spine.

1. Explain how the X-ray tube generator should be constructed to obtain cervical spine sections.

2. What parameters influence the spatial and contrast resolution of the tomographic section?

3. What type of detector is used in the design of this type of scanner? Explain its operating principle?

4. Propose the architecture of a system for acquiring 4 slices of 0.5 mm, using an asymmetrical arrangement of detectors?

5. Explain the different stages in the formation of tomographic slices acquired by a multi-slice helical scanner.

References

[1] STEVE WEBB, The contribution, history, impact and future of physics in medicine , Acta Oncologica, 48, 1772-169, 2009.

[2] DR ANTOINE GERAADS, CT scan course, January 2002.

[3] ANNIE ROUSSEAU, Physical Principles in Ultrasound, IUCPQ , September 2014.

[4] G. CALOZ, P. BOISSOLES, S. BALAC, L'Imagerie par Résonance Magnétique nucléaire, Problèmes mathématiques et numériques, Séminaire d'analyse numérique, Nantes, 2005.

[5] ZAIDI H. ED, Quantitative Analysis Of Nuclear Medicine Images, Springer, New York, 2006

[6] FLORENCE TUPIN, Introduction to image processing, OASIS Course, 2007

[7] SCHERER OLIVIER, Direction des Usages du Numérique, Ingénierie Pédagogique et Médiatisation, Université de Strasbourg, 2011.

[8] M. ÇAOUI, Bases physiques de l'imagerie médicale et de la radiothérapie, course, 2010-1011

[9] MASSON, Physique et biophysique 4, bases de l'utilisation médicale des radiations.

[10] J-P VUILLEZ, Chapitre 2 : Interactions des rayonnements avec la matière, UE3-1 : Biophysique, Université Joseph Fourier de Grenoble, 2011-2012.

[11] F. GREMY, biophysique, Flammarion 1982.

[12] D. REGENT, D. MANDRY, V. CROISE-LAURENT A. OLIVER , F. JAUSSET , V. LOMBARD, Production des rayons X en imagerie par projection et en scanographie " ,Elsevier Masson SAS. 2013.

[13] HALLIDAY, RESNICK , optics and modern physics, Renouveau Pédagogique.

[14] OLIVIER CAUDRELIER, Interaction of radiation with matter, POLY-PREPAS , Centre de Préparation aux Concours Paramédicaux

[15] D.MARIANO-GOULART, bases physiques de la radiologie pour le pcem2 , service de médecine nucléaire. chu lapeyronie. Montpellier

[16] SOLACROUP, BOYER, LE MAREC, SCHOUMAN CLAEYS, Bases physiques des rayons X, Transforamtion de l'image radiante X en image lumineuse" - CERF 2001

[17] OMAR CHERIF LEZZAR, Amplificateur de Brillance , 2010.

[18]https://fr.wikipedia.org/wiki/%C3%89cran_radioluminescent_%C3%A0_m%C3%A9moire

[19] MARTINO MICKAËL, Les Capteurs Plan, Coronary angiography department, Clinique Claude Bernard.

[20] DR. PAUL BARTHEZ, Bases Physiques et Techniques en Imagerie Médicale, TDM - IRM - D1, 2002

[21] F. DUBOIS, Reconstruction Des Images Tomographiques Par Retroprojection   Filtree, CHU Saint Etienne , Revue de l'ACOMEN, 2, vol 4,1998.

[22] DR.ENG.SARAH HAGI, CT-Generation, RAD309

[23]SOLACROUP, BOYER, LE MAREC, SCHOUMAN CLAEYS, Bases physiques des rayons X, scanner à RX, CERF 2001.

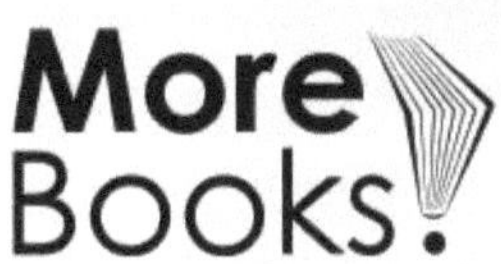

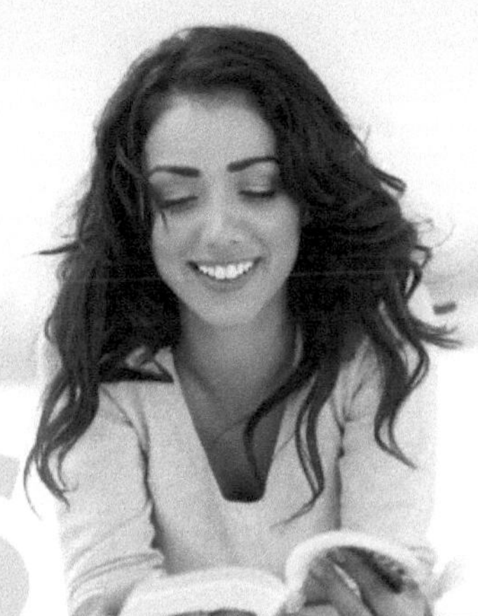

yes
I want morebooks!

Buy your books fast and straightforward online - at one of world's fastest growing online book stores! Environmentally sound due to Print-on-Demand technologies.

Buy your books online at
www.morebooks.shop

Kaufen Sie Ihre Bücher schnell und unkompliziert online – auf einer der am schnellsten wachsenden Buchhandelsplattformen weltweit! Dank Print-On-Demand umwelt- und ressourcenschonend produzi ert.

Bücher schneller online kaufen
www.morebooks.shop

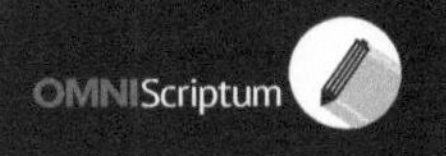

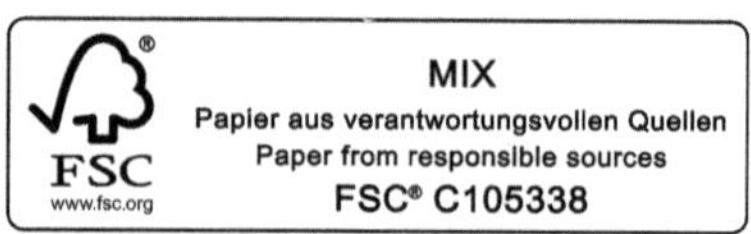

Printed by Books on Demand GmbH, Norderstedt / Germany